Leadership
in Health and Social Care
An Introduction for Emerging Leaders

Louise Jones and Clare L Bennett

Lantern

ISBN: 978 1 908625 02 1

First published in 2012 by Lantern Publishing Limited

Lantern Publishing Limited, The Old Hayloft, Vantage Business Park, Bloxham Road, Banbury OX16 9UX, UK

www.lanternpublishing.com

British Library Cataloguing in Publication Data

A catalogue record for this book is available from the British Library

The authors and publisher have made every attempt to ensure the content of this book is up to date and accurate. However, healthcare knowledge and information is changing all the time so the reader is advised to double-check any information in this text on drug usage, treatment procedures, the use of equipment, etc. to confirm that it complies with the latest safety recommendations, standards of practice and legislation, as well as local Trust policies and procedures. Students are advised to check with their tutor and/or mentor before carrying out any of the procedures in this textbook.

Cover image © Kwest – Fotolia.com

Typeset by Phoenix Photosetting, Chatham, UK

Cover design by Andrew Magee Design Ltd

Printed and bound by MPG Books Ltd, Bodmin, UK

Distributed by NBN International, 10 Thornbury Road, Plymouth, PL6 7PP, UK

CONTENTS

FOREWORD

Having been a leadership 'junkie' for many years, I am always keen to read anything new about the subject.

Whilst much of this book's content is familiar to me, I am struck by how accessible the information is and also by the fact that so much information is all in one place! For most of us, anything that saves time is of huge value.

I commend this book to you as a 'way in' to the leadership world for anyone working in health and social care. It is comprehensive and well-ordered and helps you to find out more in your own time. It treats you like an adult and *expects* you to take responsibility for your own leadership development.

This book cleverly models a leader's approach to leadership development.

We now know that good leadership has a direct relationship with good services and we can certainly no longer afford mediocrity. We need leaders to create the vision and inspire others to follow. We need leaders to enable the disruptive innovation that will be required to improve the quality of care with less resource to do so.

The inevitable tough decisions and choices that leaders will need to make mean that we need courageous leaders who have integrity and humility. My favourite quote to distinguish leaders from managers is 'Managers do things right, leaders do the right thing'.

I congratulate Louise and Clare on this publication and I hope you enjoy the journey of personal development.

Karen Middleton, Chief Health Professions Officer for England

April 2012

ABOUT THE AUTHORS

Louise Jones is a chartered physiotherapist with many years' experience in leadership roles within Higher Education and at a national level through the Chartered Society of Physiotherapy in the UK. She leads the multi-professional Institute of Health & Society at the University of Worcester, UK, and has been Vice Chair of Council at the Chartered Society of Physiotherapy.

Clare L. Bennett is a senior lecturer at the University of Worcester and has extensive experience of teaching Leadership at Foundation, Bachelors and Masters level. Clare has a special interest in Applied Leadership Studies. She has been a clinical nurse specialist in immunology and has also nursed in the fields of HIV, infectious diseases and sexual health. She is currently undertaking her Professional Doctorate in Advanced Healthcare Practice.

PREFACE

Welcome to *Leadership in Health and Social Care: An Introduction for Emerging Leaders*.

The aim of this book is to raise your awareness, knowledge and understanding of leadership issues and encourage you to start, or continue, your leadership journey. Whatever your role in health and social care, you can make a difference. However, by becoming a leader in the workplace you will be able to increase your impact and further help improve the service user experience in what is a very challenging environment.

In *Chapter 1* you will be introduced to what is meant by the term 'leadership' and why it is so important to health and social care today. In *Chapter 2* you will then start your journey along the leadership path by looking at the history and most prominent theories of leadership, so that you are able to understand the basis of leadership. Within this chapter you will have the opportunity to compare and contrast the advantages and disadvantages of different leadership styles. *Chapter 3* introduces you to the skills and qualities that make for effective leadership as well as helping you learn how you can enhance your communication skills and gain an understanding of emotional intelligence. In *Chapter 4* you will explore the cultural context in which you are working and the importance of values and beliefs as sources of motivation in addition to the relevant ethics, respect and honesty. The importance of aligning personal and organisational objectives will be considered and you will be encouraged to think about how this can be achieved. *Chapter 5* enables you to think further about the organisation in which you are working, to consider power and politics and how they impact on leadership within the organisation. You will begin to consider the different sources and bases of power and develop an understanding of the significance of symbols. You will have the opportunity to explore ways in which you can influence outcomes in the workplace and gain an understanding of how and where leadership can take place. A key element of leadership currently relates to change management and *Chapter 6* discusses what change is and helps you identify the drivers for change in your organisation. You will analyse the role of the leader as a catalyst for change and you will be introduced to change management models and the theories of motivation applied to change management. In *Chapter 7* you will gain an understanding of the structure and function of the NHS and care services in the context of how they developed and are changing in light of government policy. No health and care provider works in isolation and it is important that you appreciate the local and national context in which you are working. Service users and carers have an increasing role within health and care services and you will explore how the focus of care and focus of leadership are changing across the health and social care sector. Finally in *Chapter 8* you will look at where you go from here. The role of reflective practice in developing you as a leader will be explored and you will have the opportunity to identify your current strengths and weaknesses as a leader. You will also be encouraged to develop an action plan to address your leadership development needs.

Activities and *Scenarios* within each chapter will help you explore your own perceptions of leadership and assist you in developing strategies to enable you to unleash your potential in a realistic way within the workplace. A series of questions at the end of every chapter will help you reflect on your learning and reinforce your understanding of the key points. As well as the full reference list at the back of the book (a mixture of textbooks, articles and electronic resources) additional reading is identified at the end of each chapter which will further broaden your outlook on leadership.

Working in the health or social care environment is a great career where you can touch the lives of many. However, by developing your leadership skills you can make even more of an impact on those you work with – service users, their carers and colleagues. This is the beginning of a fantastic journey – so go unleash your potential, emerge as a leader, and make your mark in health and social care!

Louise Jones
Clare L. Bennett

April 2012

1

WHAT DO WE MEAN BY LEADERSHIP?

LEARNING OUTCOMES:

When you have completed this chapter you should be able to:

1.1 Describe what is meant by the term 'leadership'

1.2 Discuss the importance of leadership in the world of health and social care today

1.3 Recognise the different forms that leadership can take

1.4 Identify what makes a positive leadership experience.

WHAT DOES THE TERM 'LEADERSHIP' MEAN TO YOU?

The fact that you are reading this book suggests that you are interested in leadership and want to know more about being a leader. You may be a student who is about to qualify or be early in your career in health and social care but whatever the reason, this book will help you understand some of the key concepts and knowledge that will help you unleash your potential for leadership.

ACTIVITY 1.1

Identify a situation recently where you took the lead. This could be in your personal life or at work. What things did you do or say in order to 'lead'?

You may already be a leader, perhaps as captain of a sports team or youth club leader, or you may be a course representative at university or teach a class at your local sports centre. You may have taken on the role of organising a social event at work or leading a Continuing Professional Development (CPD) session as part of staff development. In any of these situations you will have enabled people to move forward together towards the same goal, not because you are forcing them to do so but because they want to. That is leadership.

Leadership skills are like any other skills; they need to be practised and refined in order to develop. Experience will shape not only the leadership skills themselves but the ways in which you use them. It will also allow you to recognise opportunities where you can take on a leadership role.

SO WHAT IS LEADERSHIP?

There are many different ways in which leadership can be, and has been, defined. What is widely recognised, however, in the simplest terms, is that in order to be a leader you have to have followers.

Rost and Barker (2000) provide us with a definition which includes influence, intention, responsibility and change, as well as the creation of a shared purpose: 'Leadership is an influence relationship among leaders and followers who intend real changes and outcomes that reflect their shared purpose'. This definition fits well with leadership in health and social care environments today.

ACTIVITY 1.2

Reflect on the place where you work or study and identify who you consider to be leaders. Write down why you think they are leaders and which part of the organisation they work in.

It is a common misconception that leaders are primarily in the top layers of an organisation; leaders can exist at all levels within organisations and society. In addition, leadership is not confined just to people working in identified leadership positions. Anyone can take the lead at some point. Jones and Jenkins (2006) identify that leadership can relate to small actions that impact on just those closest to them or much larger actions that impact on a wide range of people across, or even beyond, an organisation.

ACTIVITY 1.3

Think about what you have been doing over the past month, in your personal life or at work. Identify as many opportunities as you can where you either took the lead or had the opportunity to do so.

You may well have been surprised by the number of opportunities you identified in *Activity 1.3*, particularly by including your personal life as well as your work life. It is important to remember that many leadership skills are transferable between these two contexts.

Every experience of leadership can be different because it depends on the context as well as the skills of the person in the leadership role. However, it is very valuable for you to reflect on what makes a positive or negative experience, as this can influence how you utilise and develop your own leadership skills to ensure you are effective as a leader.

From the number of texts and articles available it is evident that leadership continues to be a source of interest to many people and it is still evolving as a discipline.

WHY IS LEADERSHIP SO IMPORTANT IN HEALTH AND SOCIAL CARE TODAY?

Health and social care has always experienced change over the years; however, the pace of change and increasing complexity of the services being delivered mean that effective leadership is more important than ever. With globalisation, society has much more social, cultural and racial diversity today and there is an increasingly ageing population who require more intervention, because long-term conditions often have more complications (Freshwater *et al.*, 2009).

Technology is becoming more advanced and affordable, and care is shifting away from institutional settings to care closer to home – for example the increasing use of telemedicine to avoid travelling to hospital. In addition, the size, shape and number of organisations involved in delivering care in the public, private and voluntary sectors has increased, such as the emergence of social enterprises and more condition-specific charities.

As a result of these changes, the approaches to care are evolving and an increasing number of different roles and functions have emerged in health and social care, such as assistant practitioner, family case worker or extended scope practitioner. This has also meant the approach to leadership has had to change, because there is a need for more leaders at all levels in order to ensure that patients and clients receive the best possible care. Instead of the strict hierarchy of previous decades, the current health and care services are less about the position or authority of an individual within an organisation and more about a leadership approach which enables effective change and enables staff to think and behave differently to bring about improvements for service users and carers. The current challenge within health and care services is to enable each individual member of staff to be actively engaged in recognising when and where they can make a leadership contribution (Jones & Jenkins, 2006).

Chapter 7 broadly considers the context in which you are, or will be, working; an understanding of which is important in order to lead effectively. It outlines the current macrostructure and functions of the National Health Service (NHS) and care services and explores how changes in government policies and the financial environment have led to new roles and ways of working within the NHS and local authorities. However, different systems and processes are in place in the four regions which make up the United Kingdom due to the devolution process, and a brief explanation of these is included. It is important to note, however, that the focus of control is moving away from the people who work in health and social care organisations to the service users who benefit from their services. For example, the Secretary of State for Health explicitly stated in 2011 that there would be 'no decision about me, without me' and this philosophy underpinned the government White Paper, *Equity and Excellence: Liberating the NHS* (Department of Health, 2010a), which proposed wide-ranging changes for both health and social care in England.

Another important factor to recognise when taking on the lead in health and social care is the increasing expectations that the public have of the health and care services. Access to the plethora of information available through the internet, including the NHS Choices website, means that people are now more informed than ever before. Service users and their carers also now expect to be treated as customers in the same way they would if they were buying a product or service in a shop or online.

ACTIVITY 1.4

Write down what you think from your experience are the pros and cons of the public's expectations of customer service from the NHS or local authorities. How might an understanding of these enable you to be a better leader?

The increasing awareness of the public in respect of health and social care issues suggests an increasing interest in their own health and wellbeing, which is really positive. However, it also creates additional challenges to those undertaking a leadership role as it changes the context in which you are working beyond the traditional boundaries of care.

INFORMAL AND FORMAL LEADERSHIP

Leadership can take many different forms, as will be discussed as you progress through this book. However, it is important to recognise that it can be both informal and formal, and that there are many different leadership styles. These will be explored in detail in *Chapter 2*.

ACTIVITY 1.5

Think about your past week and identify when you experienced either informal or formal leadership. What made these experiences different, or were they the same?

Formal leadership usually occurs in relation to a job role or position within an organisation. It may be that you are a designated team leader or key worker. These people are leaders because they are in a leadership position rather than because they necessarily have excellent leadership skills. Informal leadership tends to happen on an ad hoc basis; it may be short term, limited to the duration of a project or a particular client's care, or longer term. An example of this would be where your work colleagues turn to you and place you in a leadership role in a particular context because of your personal skills and attributes relevant to that context.

SCENARIO 1.1

June is an assistant practitioner on an orthopaedic ward where there is a rotation of staff. Because of her experience in handling this type of patient as well as her extensive knowledge of the different consultants' rehabilitation protocols, newly qualified staff and students alike look to her for guidance and support.

In this scenario, June takes on a leadership role because of the situation but also because of her level of expertise in this particular context. She is approachable and enjoys her work, which is demonstrated in the way she interacts with her patients and colleagues, and they admire her for this. However, it is an informal role rather than a positional role which is accepted by ward staff, as she is well liked and respected by her line manager and senior staff within the multidisciplinary team who recognise her skills and expertise within this area of work.

Team leadership can be both formal and informal. In many circumstances the team leader is decided upon by a line manager; however, there is an increasing use of informal groups within the health and social care sector. In these situations, when you undertake a leadership role may be less clear. Sometimes there can be consensus within the group as to who should be the leader, occurring either with or without a nomination process, and on other occasions it can be left for a leader to emerge. This form of leadership is becoming more prevalent due to the increased emphasis upon teamwork in organisations and an increasingly educated population who have their own expectations and desire to influence outcomes. An additional factor is the complexity of society where the nature of the issues to be addressed often requires a range of problem-solving skills that are seldom found in a single person (Chambers *et al.*, 2007).

Another, more informal form of leadership is becoming more apparent within health and social care. This is distributed leadership, which was originally developed within the education sector. It is seen as being the product of an interactive group or network of individuals rather than the act of a single person and it opens up the boundaries of leadership to those who would previously have been excluded from leadership activities. The underpinning principle for distributed leadership is the spreading of expertise across an organisation rather than it being concentrated on just a few people. This fits well with the concept of informal leadership mentioned above and with the comments made by Lord Darzi, about unlocking talent, in the final report of the NHS Next Stage Review, *High Quality Care for All* (Department of Health, 2008); '"unlocking talent" involves tapping into the leadership skills and potential of all frontline staff to deliver high quality, safe and effective care to patients and service users'. This fits well with the key idea that good leadership can and should exist at all levels within an organisation, and why your emergence as a leader is so valuable.

LEADERSHIP OR MANAGEMENT?

It is important to understand how leadership differs from management, since the two concepts are often confused and misunderstood (Martin *et al.*, 2010). It should be noted, however, that leadership and management often coexist in a single person, although in different ratios; leaders often need managerial skills and managers may require leadership skills. Jones and Jenkins (2006) identify leadership in action as normally being non-routine, ranging from small actions which are only noticeable to those involved in them, to significant actions which affect a much larger number of people. The differences between leadership and management are more fully explored in *Chapter 2*, which will enable you to recognise when you or your colleagues are engaging in management or leadership activities and respond appropriately. However, Schoemaker and Russo (1993) propose the comparison shown in *Table 1.1*.

Schoemaker and Russo use decision-making to draw the comparison; however, their work can also be seen to directly relate to the different roles of leadership and management. You can see why, if both leadership and management roles coexist in the same individual, they may feel some internal conflict.

ACTIVITY 1.6

Do you consider yourself currently as having opportunities to undertake more of a leadership or a management role? List the reasons why you have come to that decision.

Table 1.1 *Comparison of approaches to decision-making (Schoemaker & Russo, 1993)*

	Management	Leadership
Direction	Planning and budgeting Keeping an eye on the bottom line	Creating vision and strategy Keeping an eye on the horizon
Alignment	Organising and staffing Directing and controlling Creating boundaries	Creating shared culture and values Helping others grow Reducing boundaries
Relationships	Focusing on objects – producing or selling goods and services Based on a position of power Acting as boss	Focusing on people – inspiring and motivating followers Based on personal power Acting as coach, facilitator, servant
Personal qualities	Emotional distance Expert mind Talking Conformity Insight into organisation	Emotional connections (heart) Open mind (mindfulness) Listening (communication) Nonconformity (courage) Insight into self (integrity)
Outcomes	Maintains stability	Creates change, often radical change

WHAT MAKES A GOOD LEADER?

ACTIVITY 1.7

Think of a person you believe is an excellent leader. Write down your reasons for making this choice.

Much work has been carried out in identifying what constitutes a 'good' leader. This is focused on in more detail in *Chapter 3*. However, a key characteristic that you are likely to have identified in *Activity 1.7* is the behaviour of the leader. This is expanded upon below.

ACTIVITY 1.8

Think of two situations, either from your personal or work experience. The first situation is where a leader made a statement or promise and then acted in a highly contradictory manner. The second is where the leader followed through on their statement with positive action. Reflecting on these two situations, draw up a list of what the leaders did right and what they did wrong, and what they should have done. Now think about how you would have handled these situations. Would you have done things differently?

The behaviour of a leader can have a significant impact on the way in which a team works. It can be reflected in how motivated they are, as well as in their attitudes and values. In any group, it is the leader who has the maximum potential to sway their colleagues' emotions (Goleman *et al.*, 2009). However, it is the relationship between the leader and the team members which is the critical factor in achieving outcomes, so even when you are acting as a follower, rather than overtly taking the leadership role, you can have a positive influence on what happens. This reflects authentic leadership where the interpersonal processes between leaders and followers are pivotal. Eagly (2005) makes it clear that the relational nature of authentic leadership between leaders and followers does not rest on the efforts of the leader alone. It is a reciprocal process because leaders affect followers and vice versa.

Chambers *et al.* (2007) identify that a good leader is followed mainly because people trust and respect them. This trust and respect arise because of a number of qualities, amongst which are integrity, honesty, positivity, confidence and commitment. Good leaders develop a rapport with their team members by acting in four ways: they listen, they consult, they involve others and they explain why things need to be done as well as what needs to be done. Chambers *et al.* (2007) also argue that effective leaders are those who stick to the issues under discussion and try to minimise personal comments about individuals.

There are varying theories as to what characteristics, attributes or skills contribute to someone being considered a good leader. However, for many people the experience of being led is very personal. There are a few people whom the vast majority of observers would consider outstanding leaders, such as Martin Luther King, Jr. or Mother Teresa of Calcutta, but it is less easy within the NHS and social care in the UK to find leaders whom a whole organisation or region believes are excellent. This is because there are so many different facets to being a leader and many different perspectives from which leadership can be viewed. However, when you have reached the end of this book we hope that you will be able to identify clearly those things which contribute to successful and effective leadership and apply these to your own development.

CHAPTER SUMMARY

Three key points to take away from Chapter 1:

- ↪ Leaders can exist at all levels of the organisational hierarchy and this is reflected in the different forms that leadership can take. Leadership and management are not always linked.

- ↪ With the increasing complexity of the health and care environment, there is an increasing need for leadership in health and social care.

- ↪ Leadership can be both informal and formal. Different approaches, such as distributed leadership, will have varying degrees of success depending upon the context, but authenticity is the key.

QUESTIONS

Question 1.1

What do you understand so far by the term leadership? *(Learning outcome 1.1)*

Question 1.2

Why is leadership increasingly important in health and social care? *(Learning outcome 1.2)*

Question 1.3

What are the different forms that leadership can take? Illustrate your answer with examples from your own experience from, or outside of, work. *(Learning outcome 1.3)*

Question 1.4

What factors do you believe are important for good leadership? *(Learning outcome 1.4)*

FURTHER READING

Barr, J. & Dowding, L. (2008) *Leadership in Healthcare*. London: Sage.

Brooks, I. (2009) *Organisational Behaviour: Individuals, Groups and Organisation*, 4th edition. Harlow: Prentice Hall.

Chambers, R., Mohanna, K., Spurgeon, P. & Wall, D. (2007) *How to Succeed as a Leader*. Oxford: Radcliffe Publishing.

2

THEORIES OF LEADERSHIP

LEARNING OUTCOMES:

When you have completed this chapter you should be able to:

2.1 Outline the differences and commonalities between leadership and management

2.2 Give an overview of the history of leadership

2.3 Describe the most prominent theories of leadership

2.4 Compare the advantages and disadvantages of the different styles of leadership

2.5 Identify which leadership styles you need to develop in order to enhance your effectiveness as a leader.

INTRODUCTION

So far you have been thinking about what is meant by the term 'leadership' and the importance of leadership in health and social care today. You have also been considering the different forms leadership can take. You have related this to your own experiences of leadership and you have identified why some leadership encounters may be more positive than others. This chapter moves on to examine the key theories that underpin leadership today and will inform your analysis further. It starts by delineating leadership and management. It then goes on to consider the history of leadership and leadership theory. The various styles of leadership are then critically examined to help you to develop an awareness of the various leadership styles and how these can be applied to your daily work. The discussions and activities will help you to apply the theories to your personal and professional development as a leader.

ARE YOU A LEADER OR A MANAGER?

ACTIVITY 2.1

'Management and leadership are the same' [quote from first-year student nurse]

Do you agree with this opinion? Justify your answer, identifying any differences and similarities between leadership and management.

There is much confusion surrounding the distinction between leadership and management, with the two terms often being used interchangeably. In practice, many 'managers' will have leadership roles and many 'leaders' will have managerial responsibilities, which exacerbates the confusion. However, in order for practitioners to flourish in these respective roles, leadership and management need to be viewed as two distinct concepts (Stanley, 2006).

ACTIVITY 2.2

Make a list of activities that you or your colleagues engage in when you are 'managing' and those that are undertaken when 'leading'.

Your list of management activities will probably have been largely concerned with operational issues such as planning, resource management and problem solving, as these are roles that characterise managerial responsibilities. Managerial activities are essential to the smooth running of any organisation and the attainment of care standards and targets. They are not, therefore, secondary in importance to leadership roles, as is sometimes perceived (Iles, 2006).

Watson (1983) uses the 'seven Ss' model to differentiate between managerial and leadership roles. The model proposes that managers rely on strategy, structure and systems, whereas leaders use the 'softer' Ss – staff, style, shared goals and skills.

Unlike management, leadership is not related to seniority within an organisation. It is largely concerned with working towards or positively adapting to change (Parks, 2005). Leadership activities are generally centred on providing the vision and inspiration to enable groups of people to work together towards the achievement of a common goal.

ACTIVITY 2.3

Identify situations where you have seen leadership, as described above, in action. What skills did the leader use in order to convey his or her vision?

As outlined in *Chapter 3*, individuals will possess different leadership skills and qualities which will inform your response to *Activity 2.3*. Other issues that will influence the way in which leaders convey their message will be less obvious, in that they centre on the individual's attitudes and beliefs about their role as a leader and the style(s) which they use in different contexts. These issues will now be explored.

THE HISTORY OF LEADERSHIP

The last century has seen 'leadership' examined, analysed and debated by a host of social scientists, resulting in a plethora of leadership theories. At the time of writing, a commercial search engine for books listed in excess of 170 280 leadership titles and an academic search engine for articles focusing on leadership listed 87 944!

Due to the complexities and varying contexts of leadership there is no single theory that fully explains what leadership is and what aspects of leadership work best. This chapter therefore examines the theories that are of most relevance to health and social care today. Each set of theories is examined in chronological order. As you will see, the emphasis shifts throughout the decades to reflect events of the time, society's expectations and the prevailing mood (McKimm & Held, 2009). Whilst each theory has its limitations, aspects will still be of use today.

DEFINING 'THEORY'

ACTIVITY 2.4

What does the term 'theory' mean to you? Compare your definition with dictionary definitions on the internet.

A theory provides a testable framework for describing some aspect of the natural world. It is supported by evidence from repeated observation and testing and incorporates facts, laws, predictions and tested hypotheses. Leadership theory originates from psychology, sociology, organisational science and political science. It aims to provide a model for understanding leadership behaviours and their predicted impact.

THE TRAIT THEORIES

ACTIVITY 2.5

Using the template below, write a job description for the perfect leader.

Job description

Job title: Leader

Job purpose:

Main responsibilities:

Essential qualities:

The essential qualities that you identified in the job description are likely to have been underpinned by the trait approach to leadership. This is sometimes referred to as *constitutional theory*. Although trait theory is one of the earliest perspectives on leadership, it is still relevant today. Trait theories are concerned with the necessary personal qualities, physical abilities and personality traits that characterise an effective leader. Throughout the late nineteenth century and the early part of the twentieth century, leadership theorists asserted that leaders were born, not made, which gave rise to the 'Great Man' theories (Galton, 1869, cited in Morrison, 1993). The theories originated from the study of celebrated social, political and military leaders throughout history and the identification of innate qualities that characterised these people. The belief was that only certain 'great' people were born with these traits (Northouse, 2010).

In a significant review of leadership theory at that time Stogdill (1948) identified eight traits that distinguished leaders from followers:

- intelligence

- alertness

- insight

- responsibility

- initiative

- persistence

- self-confidence

- sociability

Since this time many theorists have attempted to investigate further the traits that underpin successful leaders, as will be shown in *Chapter 3*. However, as yet no definitive list of essential leadership traits exists. Leaders will naturally exhibit different qualities and there are many great leaders who do not possess all of the traits identified by trait theories over the decades (Gopee & Galloway, 2009).

In his review of the leadership literature spanning the period 1904–1947 Stogdill (1948) argued that no single specific set of traits could consistently differentiate leaders from followers. He also suggested that the success of a leader may depend upon the specific leadership context; a leader with leadership traits may be successful in one situation but enjoy less success in other leadership situations. This perspective represented a significant challenge to trait theory which had previously implied that if leaders possessed leadership traits they would be able to lead all people in all situations. In identifying an interaction between the leader, people and context Stogdill's (1948) review of the literature signalled a change in focus from the traits of a leader to the wider context of leadership. Consequently, the emphasis of leadership research changed to a focus on leadership behaviours and leadership situations (Northouse, 2010).

ACTIVITY 2.6

Based on what you have read so far, do you feel that trait theory is still of relevance today, despite its limitations? Or should it be disregarded as fundamentally flawed?

Although there are many valid criticisms of trait theory, the trait approach to leadership has recently re-emerged with the increased interest in charismatic leadership styles (Northouse, 2010). Many of the qualities outlined by trait theorists are still used to describe successful leaders today. For example, when looking at descriptions of Nelson Mandela, the former President of South Africa, traits such as 'inspirational', 'stoic' and 'moral' are frequently referred to in commentaries and analyses. As McKimm and Held (2009) point out, certain qualities of the 'hero leader' such as tenacity and intelligence are arguably as necessary and relevant today as they have ever been. In health and social care this is borne out by the number of studies currently focusing on leadership qualities. For example, Littlewood and Strozier (2009) have recently carried out a study that explores and measures leadership qualities in grandparents and other relatives raising children. In nursing, Zilembo and Monterosso (2008) published work which describes nursing students' perceptions of desirable leadership qualities in nurse preceptors. In sport, Tucker (2010) has carried out an analysis of sports coaches' leadership qualities and their impact on male and female athletes in middle schools.

ACTIVITY 2.7

Carry out a literature search for articles that focus on leadership qualities in your field of work. How many did you find? What does this say about the relevance of trait theory in health and social care today?

THE BEHAVIOURAL THEORIES

The behavioural theories, sometimes referred to as the *circumstantial theories* or *style approach*, focus on the behaviour of leaders. They suggest that leaders are engaged in two specific sets of behaviour: task-focused behaviours and relationship-focused behaviours (Blake & Mouton, 1964). Task-focused behaviours are concerned with facilitating the achievement of objectives. Relationship-focused behaviours are centred on inter-personal relationships and helping individuals and teams feel comfortable with the work situation (Northouse, 2010). The focus of the styles approach is on how leaders integrate these two sets of behaviours and adjust their behaviour in response to the specific context (Blake & Mouton, 1964; McKimm & Held, 2009). A more task-focused approach may be necessary in one context, such as an emergency, whereas a more relationship-focused approach may be appropriate in another situation, such as the management of change.

Action-centred leadership

Adair's model of action-centred leadership (Adair, 2009) asserts that there are three principal areas of need in a working group:

- The task needs, i.e. the need to achieve the joint objective or goal

- The team maintenance needs, i.e. the need to be held together as an effective team

- The individual needs, i.e. the human needs of each individual.

The model is presented as three overlapping circles that demonstrate the distinctive nature of each need along with the inter-dependence of the three areas.

ACTIVITY 2.8

Jane is a manager of a prison healthcare unit. A recent audit has revealed that the level of hepatitis B vaccination taken up by prisoners is well below the desired standard. She needs her team to increase the level of hepatitis B vaccination amongst prisoners. Apply the three areas of need outlined by Adair (2009) (task needs, team maintenance needs and individual needs) to this case study, using the three overlapping circles outlined below.

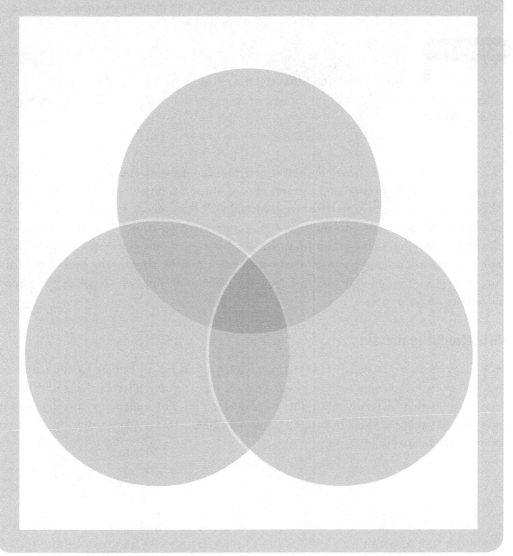

The leader's role is to facilitate the team in meeting these needs and managing tensions that may arise from conflicting areas of need. This requires a 'functional approach' to leadership which involves the leader in areas such as clarifying the task, planning, evaluating, motivating and role-modelling. In order to increase the level of hepatitis B vaccination amongst prisoners, the *task needs* that may need to be addressed could include identifying ways in which the goal can be achieved, for example, by identifying times when the issue of hepatitis B vaccination can be raised with prisoners, and the implementation of vaccination clinics. The *team maintenance needs* will be concerned with issues such as clear communication between team members to ensure that everyone is clear about their role within the project, the direction the project is taking and motivation. In addressing *individual needs*, issues such as the need for training and education may be addressed along with ensuring that individuals feel able to address any questions or concerns that they may have.

ACTIVITY 2.9

Return to the overlapping circles that you have filled in for *Activity 2.8*. If you completely shade out one of the circles, what impact does this have on the remaining two circles?

Activity 2.9 emphasises the strength of the relationship between the three needs identified in Adair's model. By overlooking one area of need, the remaining two areas can be adversely affected. In order to provide effective leadership all three needs have to be met. If, for example, the prison healthcare manager concentrates all of her efforts on setting up hepatitis B vaccination clinics and maximising the number of patients vaccinated in each clinic, but neglects to encourage and motivate staff, there may be short-term gains but in the longer term motivation and job satisfaction are likely to decline, which is likely to impact negatively on outcomes.

Situational leadership

For many years it was widely believed that leaders could rigidly adhere to one particular leadership style and enjoy success. However, more recent research has challenged this view and suggests that leaders who are able to adapt their style of leadership to each situation and context are more likely to succeed (Goleman, 2000). This is a key characteristic of the *contingency* theories of leadership.

ACTIVITY 2.10

Before discussing how the various leadership styles can be matched to the needs of the individual and situation it is important that you check your understanding of some of the key leadership styles. Test your understanding of the following leadership styles by describing them and analysing how they are likely to impact on a team's performance.

Leadership style	Description	Potential impact on team performance
Autocratic		
Bureaucratic		
Charismatic		
Democratic		
Laissez-faire		

Autocratic leadership is characterised by a lack of consultation with colleagues, a desire for control in decision-making and limited delegation. An autocratic approach can be desirable in a crisis situation where clear direction and quick decision-making are required. However, if the autocratic style is employed long term it is likely to lead to a lack of motivation, reduced job satisfaction and low morale.

Bureaucratic leadership styles are concerned with ensuring that staff follow rules, policies and procedures accurately and consistently. As a result, practices are safe and standards are maintained. However, this style can stifle creativity and autonomy, resulting in demotivated staff and an organisation that does not move forward.

Charismatic leadership styles rely on the behaviours and qualities of the leader. The key behaviours of the charismatic leader include an ability to inspire, the setting of high expectations and development of a collective identity. The success of this leadership style depends very much upon the perceptions of the followers. If their values are consistent with those of the leader and they seek personal growth, they are more likely to identify with the leader. Charismatic leadership can, however, also take negative forms if the leader's motives are concerned with benefit to self and the emphasis is on control.

Democratic leadership promotes the sharing of responsibility, consultation, delegation and feedback. A culture of leadership development is also evident. Benefits include enhanced decision-making, open communication and a motivated workforce that feels valued. The drawbacks are lengthy decision-making processes which can cause frustration and incur high costs.

The laissez-faire *approach* to leadership is characterised by the leader providing little or no direction, giving employees ultimate freedom. All authority is given to staff; they must establish goals, make decisions and resolve problems on their own. This can be an effective style to use when staff are highly experienced, competent and motivated. However, it can be overwhelming and unsafe if staff feel insecure and if no feedback is given.

ACTIVITY 2.11

Outline situations when each of the above leadership styles may be appropriate.

Situational leadership theory

Hersey and Blanchard's theory of situational leadership (Hersey *et al.*, 1996) asserts that leadership styles are best assessed for their suitability for the context in which they are used. In other words, there is no single 'best style' for a leader because the 'best style' will depend upon the demands of the situation. Situational leadership theory promotes the notion that leaders are responsible for fostering growth and development of themselves as well as others. It also asserts that leaders require sufficient self-awareness to appreciate when they need to let others lead, and become the 'follower'. An example of this may be when a newly qualified member of the team assumes leadership responsibility for a certain area of practice of which he or she is particularly knowledgeable.

Situational leadership theory focuses on 'follower maturity', which describes the ability and willingness of individuals to take responsibility for directing their own behaviour. This will depend upon both the individual's job maturity in relation to their knowledge, ability and experience as well as their psychological maturity in terms of how self-motivated they are. Followers are described on a continuum of 'follower readiness', as outlined in *Table 2.1*. The individual's readiness level (R) may vary across the various aspects of their role. For example, a dietitian may be at R4 in providing nutritional advice for people who have type 1 diabetes, but may be inexperienced in teaching patients about insulin pumps and is therefore at R2 for this aspect of their role. People's readiness levels may also change over time; for example, a physiotherapist may have been operating at R4 but has suffered a loss of confidence following extended sickness absence, reducing their readiness level to R3.

Table 2.1 *Four levels of follower readiness (R – 'readiness level')*

R1: Unable and unwilling or insecure; neither confident nor competent (low readiness).
R2: Unable but willing or motivated; confident but incompetent (moderate readiness).
R3: Able but unwilling or insecure; competent but unconfident or unmotivated (moderate readiness).
R4: Able and willing, competent and confident or motivated (high readiness).

Hersey *et al.* (1996) identify four leadership styles (see *Table 2.2*) that vary in the amount of direction and support the leader provides and how much involvement the follower has in decision-making regarding how work should be completed. The theory proposes that the readiness level of an individual should be matched with the appropriate leadership style. R1 will require a directional style (I), R2 will be best met by a coaching style (II), R3 requires support (III) and R4 is best served through delegation (IV).

Table 2.2 *Leadership styles*

I:	Directing
II:	Coaching
III:	Supporting
IV:	Delegating

ACTIVITY 2.12

Identify examples of how the readiness levels outlined in *Table 2.1* could be matched with the leadership styles outlined in *Table 2.2*. What are the strengths and weaknesses of this approach?

A real strength of this model is that it highlights the dynamic relationship between leaders and followers, in that it emphasises how each group and individual will require a different approach from their leader in response to differing contexts. It also draws attention to the need for leaders to accurately assess their staff in terms of their competence and confidence within the varying facets of their roles, in order that their needs can best be met.

Limitations of the model centre on the need for an accurate assessment and diagnosis of the individual's readiness level. There is no diagnostic instrument to assist this process and errors could easily occur. Limitations in the leader's listening and observation skills as well as emotional intelligence could potentially lead to a flawed judgement and therefore an inappropriate style of leadership. Additional issues associated with assessing the readiness levels of individuals and groups include the amount of time this takes in practice and also how tiring this may be for the leader. Finally, some leaders may find it challenging to adapt their behaviours so readily.

Despite these limitations, more recent work by Goleman (2000) lends further support to situational leadership theory. Goleman asserts that the most effective leaders do not rely on only one leadership style; instead they adapt their style or styles according to the specific situation and people involved. In supporting this assertion, Goleman cites a study which used a random sample of 3871 executives with the aim of identifying what underpins 'effective leadership'. The study identified six distinct leadership styles which appear to directly impact, positively or negatively, on the working atmosphere of the company, department or team. A relationship between the impact of specific leadership styles on the emotional climate of the organisation and the organisation's financial performance was also identified. This is illustrated in *Figure 2.1*.

Leadership style		Leadership behaviour		Impact on atmosphere and performance
Coercive	⇨	Demands instant compliance	⇨	Negative – people resist
Authoritative	⇨	Moves people towards a vision	⇨	Positive
Affiliative	⇨	Creates harmony and emotional attachments	⇨	Positive
Democratic	⇨	Fosters consensus through participation	⇨	Positive
Pacesetting	⇨	Expects very high standards and initiative	⇨	Negative – people become overwhelmed and demotivated
Coaching	⇨	Invests in people for the future	⇨	Positive

Figure 2.1 *The six styles of leadership (Goleman, 2000)*

ACTIVITY 2.13

What do you feel your natural or preferred leadership style is? What impact do you think this has on your colleagues? Based on your reading so far, are there any other leadership styles you feel would enhance your ability to lead?

NEW PARADIGM LEADERSHIP THEORIES

Categorising leadership theories chronologically is problematic, as many of the original leadership theories are still of relevance today. However, it is largely accepted that the more recent approaches are referred to as contemporary or new paradigm theories. The new paradigm leadership theories that will be covered in this section include transactional, transformational and servant leadership.

Transactional leadership

Transactional leadership assumes that people are motivated by reward and punishment. It is built around the notion of reciprocity, where the relationship between the leader and follower is based on the exchange of some reward, such as pay, recognition or praise. The transactional leader works through creating clear structures and clarifying goals and objectives to ensure that wider organisational goals are met. Such a relationship depends on the assumption that people are largely motivated by money and simple reward, and their behaviour is therefore predictable. However, such an assumption overlooks the complex social and emotional factors that underpin many people's motivation, as will be examined in *Chapter 6*.

For many years transactional leadership has been disregarded as a rather dated, old-fashioned management approach to leadership. However, more recent analysis has recognised the merits of transactional leadership when used alongside other leadership approaches (Bass, 1985). For example, the Head of Occupational Therapy may need to use transactional approaches in order to achieve specific key performance indicators, but may use the transformational approach, outlined in the following section, in order to bring about new ways of working. The introduction of payment systems within the NHS that reward or penalise organisations for the achievement or non-achievement of targets has also led to more transactional approaches to leadership throughout the NHS.

Transformational leadership

The transformational approach to leadership was outlined by Downton (1973), Burns (1978) and Bass (1985, 1990). It emerged from efforts to differentiate between management that was associated with transactional leadership and leadership that was focused on developing the individual.

Transformational leadership is concerned with engaging the hearts and minds of staff. It aims to help individuals and groups achieve greater motivation, satisfaction and a sense of achievement. It is based on the assumption that people will follow those who inspire them. Transformational leadership starts with the development of a vision, a view of the future that will inspire potential followers. The vision is then 'sold' to the followers and ways forward are developed. The leader is highly visible throughout and leads through example. Trust, concern and facilitation rather than direct control are key characteristics of this approach. Whilst charisma may help the leader in conveying their message, this is certainly not the only quality required. An ability to empower people, coaching, investing in others and challenging the culture to change are all necessary qualities and skills. In transformational leadership, the power of the leader comes from creating understanding and trust. The transformational leader can operate at every level within the organisational hierarchy (Stanley, 2009). This is in contrast to transactional leadership where power is associated with hierarchy and position.

Transformational leadership is widely held to be suited to leadership in care-related fields where change is constant (Welford, 2002; Thyer, 2003; NHS Confederation, 1999). The NHS Leadership Qualities Framework (NHS Institute for Innovation and Improvement, 2005a), outlined in *Figure 3.2* on page 32, was designed around this approach to leadership. However, Bass (1985) argues that transformational leadership alone is not adequate if it is not combined with transactional methods of leadership. This is particularly salient to health and social care today, with the need to attain key performance indicators.

Servant leadership

Servant leadership is based on the premise that the individual wishes to serve others first and then a conscious choice is made that one aspires to lead (Greenleaf, 1970). It is underpinned by altruistic principles that include a responsibility on the part of the leader for the followers and towards society and those who are disadvantaged. The servant leader serves others by helping them achieve and improve, rather than others serving the leader.

The principles of servant leadership defined by the Alliance for Servant Leadership (2010) include: transformation, personal growth, enabling environments, service, trusting relationships, creating commitment, community building and nurturing the spirit.

McKimm and Held (2009) discuss servant leadership in the context of 'public service'. They contend that the public services, which encompass health and social care, are primarily focused towards serving the needs of patients and clients within ethical, professional frameworks, rather than meeting the needs of the professionals delivering the service. Howatson-Jones (2004) also argues that servant leadership is applicable to the NHS with particular reference to nursing, in that it reflects the ethos of nursing and government policy for the NHS. She argues that trust and empathy help to clarify expectations and sustain change and growth.

However, a survey by Walker *et al.* (2005) suggests that the concept of servant leadership can be associated with being a slave to someone else and equated with passivity and de-powered leadership. It was also felt by some respondents to be limited in its application, for example in crisis situations. Concern was also expressed that it could lead to burnout amongst leaders because the servant leader puts aside concern for self.

IDENTIFYING YOUR LEADERSHIP STYLE

Throughout this chapter you may have identified with certain leadership styles more than others. Intuitively you may be aware of your preferred leadership style. The following activity is designed to prompt you further in identifying the leadership styles which you are comfortable with and those that you may wish to develop further.

ACTIVITY 2.14

Imagine the following scenario:

You have volunteered to lead a project with a team of seven colleagues which aims to enhance the quality of feedback that your organisation receives from patients and clients. You have outlined the aims of the project and everyone seems to understand. You have also allowed the team to get to know one another. However, when you ask the team for initial ideas they repeatedly fall quiet.

What would you do? What type of leadership style would you use? Are there any other styles that have been addressed in this chapter that you could use?

The team get over this first hurdle and begin to work productively. They come up with numerous ideas, but they do not address a point which you feel is essential: service user involvement.

How would you handle this? Would you tell the team directly? Would you not intervene? Would you try to direct the discussions towards this point? What does your answer tell you about your chosen style? What are the potential benefits and drawbacks of this style? Is there another style that may be more productive in this situation?

A decision now needs to be made about how the patient satisfaction survey could be better presented. Two of your colleagues have emerged as very strong leaders and they are knowledgeable of the field. They make two contrasting suggestions and both try to take the lead with their suggestion.

As the formal leader, what leadership style would you use in this situation? What are the likely outcomes of using this style?

This example illustrates the breadth of leadership styles that you may be required to use in any single leadership situation. As you develop your leadership skills you will become more adept at altering your leadership style to the needs of the situation. This requires much thought and practice. This theme will be built upon throughout the following chapters and will be revisited in the final chapter.

CHAPTER SUMMARY

Three key points to take away from Chapter 2:

- 'Leadership' and 'management', whilst of equal importance to the success of an organisation, differ in their focus. Management is more concerned with operational issues, whereas leadership is centred on providing vision and inspiration to enable teams to attain a common goal.

- Current leadership theory suggests that whilst some leadership qualities may be innate, they can also be developed and learnt.

- No single best leadership theory prevails. Instead, the requirements of the specific situation have to be assessed and matched with the leadership style that best meets the needs of the individual or team in that particular context.

QUESTIONS

Question 2.1

Is there a difference between leadership and management? If there is a difference, what is it? *(Learning outcome 2.1)*

Question 2.2

What was the most prominent leadership theory in the early part of the twentieth century? How have beliefs about leadership developed since this time? *(Learning outcome 2.2)*

Question 2.3

Make a list of the leadership theories that you have read about in this chapter and write three bullet points summarising them. *(Learning outcome 2.3)*

Question 2.4

What are the advantages and disadvantages of the autocratic, bureaucratic, charismatic, democratic and *laissez-faire* leadership styles? *(Learning outcome 2.4)*

Question 2.5

Which leadership styles do you need to develop in order to enhance your effectiveness as a leader? *(Learning outcome 2.5)*

FURTHER READING

Adair, J. (2009) *Not Bosses But Leaders. How to Lead the Way to Success*, 3rd edition. London: Kogan Page.

Goleman, D. (2000) Leadership that gets results. *Harvard Business Review*, **72(2):** 78–90.

Northouse, P.G. (2010) *Leadership: Theory and Practice.* London: Sage.

3

THE SKILLS AND QUALITIES OF EFFECTIVE LEADERS

LEARNING OUTCOMES:

When you have completed this chapter you should be able to:

3.1 Discuss whether leaders are born or whether they are made

3.2 Outline the key skills of an effective leader

3.3 Debate the most important qualities of a leader

3.4 Describe methods of enhancing communication

3.5 Demonstrate an understanding of emotional intelligence.

INTRODUCTION

The previous two chapters have been concerned with clarifying what we mean by leadership and providing an overview of the various leadership theories. In this chapter we consider factors that make a leader successful and how leadership qualities and skills impact on followers' behaviours.

Goffee and Jones (2000) spent ten years asking leaders 'Why should anyone be led by you?' to be met by bewildered silence. This chapter aims to help you develop some key leadership qualities and skills so that you will be able to answer this question.

ARE LEADERS BORN OR MADE?

ACTIVITY 3.1

Is leadership learned or innate? Use a mind map® to explore your thoughts. If you have not used a mind map previously, *Figure 3.1* will be helpful. In addition, you may find it useful to read Tony Buzan's work in this field (see *'Further Reading'* at the end of this chapter).

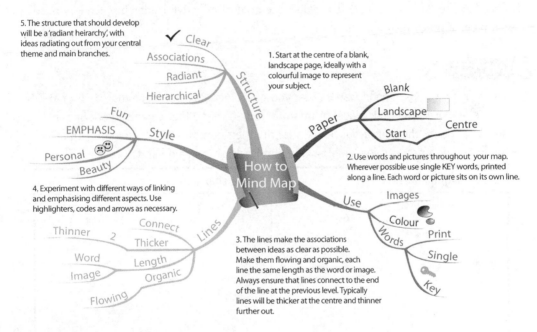

Figure 3.1 *How to make a Mind Map (Illumine, 2010). Reproduced with permission from Illumine Training.*

For centuries people have debated whether leaders are born or made. There is a group of 'trait' theories in the leadership literature that we have already referred to in *Chapter 2*. They are concerned with the necessary qualities and traits that characterise an effective leader. One group of these theories is the 'Great Man' theories which assert that some people are born to lead and others are born to be led (Galton, 1869, cited in Morrison, 1993). The Great Man theories originate from the study of great social, political and military leaders throughout history and the identification of innate qualities that characterised these people. The belief was that only certain 'great' people were born with these traits (Northouse, 2010).

Later research in the mid-twentieth century, however, questioned this belief and the emphasis began to centre more on interactions and relationships between leaders and followers, as well as on the impact that specific situations and contexts may have on the leader–follower relationship (Bernhard & Walsh, 2006). It was found that people may be great leaders in one situation but be less effective in others (Stogdill, 1948). It was also found that many leadership qualities can be developed over time (Mumford *et al.*, 2000).

WHAT ARE THE KEY SKILLS AND QUALITIES OF A LEADER?

Leadership is principally concerned with human relationships and dynamics. When done well, leadership can motivate people to perform to exceptional levels and achieve great things (Goffee & Jones, 2009). To realise the goal of effective leadership, leaders need to develop certain key qualities and skills.

ACTIVITY 3.2

Think of examples of good leaders that you have encountered; these may be formal (e.g. a leader in the work place) or informal (e.g. a friend that organised and led a holiday). Using the grid layout below, identify their qualities and their skills. What is the difference between leadership skills and leadership qualities?

Leadership qualities	Leadership skills

Leadership qualities are concerned with the attitudes and behaviours that characterise a person. Sometimes these are termed 'human qualities'. Leadership skills refer to knowledge and methods of working. These too will impact on leadership behaviour.

Leadership qualities

Maxwell (1999) outlines 21 'indispensable' qualities of a leader:

Table 3.1 *Maxwell's indispensable qualities of a leader (Maxwell, 1999)*

Character	Focus	Relationships
Charisma	Generosity	Responsibility
Commitment	Initiative	Security
Communication	Listening	Self-discipline
Competence	Passion	Servanthood
Courage	Positive attitude	Teachability
Discernment	Problem solving	Vision

ACTIVITY 3.3

Consider how important each of these qualities are by ranking the four that you consider most important from 1 (the most important) to 4 (the least important). Justify your answer.

To identify key leadership qualities that are pertinent specifically to the NHS, the NHS Institute for Innovation and Improvement (2005a) carried out an analysis of 150 chief executives and directors, with validation from other public and private sector organisations. From these data the NHS Leadership Qualities Framework (NHS Institute for Innovation and Improvement, 2005a) was designed. *Figure 3.2* outlines the 15 key leadership qualities that the analyses revealed, arranged in three core areas of leadership: *Setting Direction*; *Delivering Services* and *Personal Qualities*.

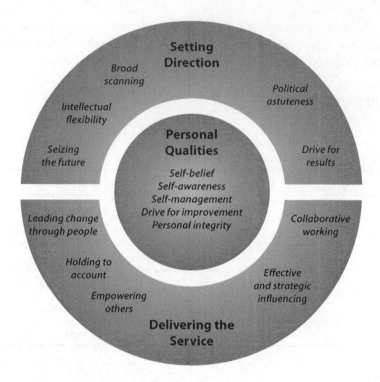

Figure 3.2 *NHS Leadership Qualities Framework (NHS Institute for Innovation and Improvement, 2005a). Reproduced with permission from NHS Institute for Innovation and Improvement.*

Personal Qualities are at the centre of the framework. These encompass:

- 'self-belief' characterised by a positive 'can do' sense of confidence

- 'self-awareness' in relation to strengths and limitations, emotions and their impact on others

- 'self-management' including the ability to regulate mood and behaviour

- 'drive for improvement' which is demonstrated by a clear focus on achievement of goals for the greater good of others

- 'personal integrity' which refers to values, openness and resilience (NHS Institute for Innovation and Improvement, 2006).

Setting Direction is concerned with:

- 'seizing the future' which describes the motivation to take transformational action and exploit opportunities to bring about improvements and political awareness

- 'intellectual flexibility' in being able to see both the bigger picture and intricate detail, having a receptiveness to different perspectives and an openness to innovative thinking

- 'broad scanning' characterised by networking and keeping abreast of local and national developments

- 'political astuteness' in terms of understanding the climate and culture of the organisation as well as the national context; understanding who the key influencers are and an awareness of health strategy and policy

- 'drive for results' in relation to the motivation to transform services, the setting of ambitious targets and actively seeking out opportunities to improve delivery of service (NHS Institute for Innovation and Improvement, 2006).

Delivering the Service involves:

- 'leading change through people' by articulating the vision clearly; keeping the focus on change and inspiring others

- 'holding to account' by setting clear targets and standards; creating a climate of support and accountability and holding people to account for what they have agreed to deliver

- 'empowering others' by allowing others to take the lead when appropriate; supporting the development of others and ensuring equality of opportunity

- 'effective and strategic influencing' by working in partnership both within the organisation and externally and employing a range of influencing strategies

- 'collaborative working' through ensuring that the strategy for health improvement, and the planning, development and provision of health services, are cohesive and 'joined up' (NHS Institute for Innovation and Improvement, 2006).

Skills for Care have carried out a mapping exercise of leadership and management standards for social care (McDonnell & Zutshi, 2005) to underpin the Skills for Care Leadership and Management Strategy (Skills for Care, 2008). These incorporate the NHS Leadership Qualities Framework (NHS Institute for Innovation and Improvement, 2005a) and the NHS Knowledge and Skills Framework (Department of Health, 2003a). They outline six functional areas or standards:

- Managing self and personal skills

- Providing direction

- Facilitating change

- Working with people

- Using resources

- Achieving results.

Look back at the leadership qualities outlined by the NHS Leadership Qualities Framework and Skills for Care. Identify any qualities that you feel you need to develop in order to enhance your leadership performance both now and in the future.

Should leaders appear human?

Goffee and Jones's work (2000) supports the assertion that effective leaders require vision, energy, authority and strategic direction. However, they go on to argue that inspirational leaders also share an additional four qualities:

- They choose, at appropriate times, to show their weaknesses. By selectively exposing their vulnerability, they can enhance how others perceive them in terms of coming across as approachable and human.

- They use intuition to gauge the timing and course of their actions. They collect and use soft data, concerned with people's emotions, to help them identify when and how to act.

- They empathise fully, yet realistically, with people and they care passionately about the work their followers do.

- They show and capitalise on what makes them unique.

Goffee and Jones (2000) assert that, to be truly inspirational, leaders need all four qualities; with one or two qualities rarely being sufficient. Inspirational leaders tend to match the most appropriate qualities to demonstrate with the style required by each particular context. For this approach to be successful, however, the leader must remain authentic.

Leadership skills

Northouse (2010) defines leadership skills as:

> 'the ability to use one's knowledge and competencies to accomplish a set of goals or objectives'. (Northouse, 2010, p. 40)

Visualise where you would like to be in your career in five years' time. Where would you like to be in 10 years' time? What leadership skills will you need in order to realise these achievements?

Katz's work in the 1950s is seminal to the skills approach to leadership (Katz, 1955). His work aimed to address leadership in terms of three sets of skills that can be developed: technical, human and conceptual; asserting that although the significance of each skill may vary depending on the leader's position within the organisation, each skill is still important for successful leaders to possess.

Technical skills are concerned with knowledge, proficiency and competence in a specific field of work or activity. They also refer to analytical capabilities and the ability to use specialist tools and techniques (Katz, 1955). Technical skills are more important at the lower levels of the organisational hierarchy (Goleman, 1998a; Katz, 1955).

Katz (1955) defined human skills as 'the ability to work effectively as a group member and to build cooperative effort within the team ...' (Katz, 1955, p. 34). Human skills are characterised by how a leader consistently perceives and behaves towards superiors, peers, and followers. Leaders engage in human skills when they motivate individuals and groups, demonstrate empathy and understanding and involve others in decision-making. Human skills are essential throughout all levels of leadership (Hicks & Gullett, 1975; Katz, 1955).

Conceptual skills encompass the 'thinking skills' needed by leaders. This set of skills involves being able to see both the bigger picture in terms of what is going on within the entire organisation, as well as the organisation in terms of its component parts and how they interact and depend on one another (Katz, 1955). Conceptual skills are likely to be of most value at the higher levels of the organisational hierarchy where policy decisions and long-term actions are required (Hicks & Gullett, 1975; Katz, 1955).

More recently Mumford *et al.* (2000) have advanced this work further to develop a skill-based model of leadership. The model examines the relationship between leadership performance and the individual leader's knowledge and skills. It is asserted that leadership qualities can be developed over time through education, training and experience.

The model is based on the belief that leadership is dependent upon the individual's ability to develop and implement appropriate solutions to complex problems. The individual's capacity to problem solve will depend upon:

- *complex problem solving skills,* which are concerned with identifying and understanding the problem and developing potential solutions;

- *social judgement skills,* which involve refining potential solutions and creating ways of implementing solutions within complex organisations;

- *social skills,* which relate to the ability to motivate and direct others during the implementation of solutions.

Shaun has been qualified as a nurse for 12 months and works as a District Nurse. He has noticed consistent time delays between patients being discharged from hospital and the first visit made by the District Nursing Team to the patient's home. Shaun wants to lead on a project which improves this situation.

Identify the knowledge that Shaun may require to successfully lead this project.

Application of *complex problem solving skills*, *social judgement skills* and *social skills* is associated with various forms of knowledge, such as an understanding of the organisation and its processes and an understanding of people, particularly those who will be instrumental in implementing solutions. As with skills, knowledge is believed to develop with experience (Mumford *et al.*, 2000). Mumford *et al.* (2000) assert that without knowledge, the skills outlined above are not adequate for effective leadership, as knowledge is essential to a leader's ability to define and solve complex organisational problems.

In Shaun's case (*Scenario 3.1*) knowledge will be required of the current processes involved in the referral system from hospital staff to the district nursing team; for example, the methods of communication involved, working patterns of both teams and identification of flaws in the current processes. These areas of knowledge will underpin the *complex problem solving skills* required by Shaun as a leader. Knowledge that is relevant to *social judgement skills* will relate to an understanding of potential solutions that will resolve the issue; for example, changes in shift patterns, job roles and methods of communication. A knowledge of human resources regulations, job descriptions and the availability of funding for additional telephones, IT resources and staff may also be required. With regard to *social skills*, an understanding of the people involved within both teams will enable Shaun to be more productive in motivating and directing others towards a change in practice.

COMMUNICATING EFFECTIVELY

Effective communication has been demonstrated to be a key attribute of clinical leaders (Stanley, 2009).

What is effective communication?

Communication is concerned with a set of interchanges that occur between individuals and groups to both give and receive information (Gopee & Galloway, 2009). Communication can be both verbal and non-verbal.

ACTIVITY 3.6

Outline what effective communication means to you. Next, think of two people communicating and consider all the simultaneous events that occur within that interaction. You may wish to consider non-verbal communication, people's perceptions of each other (based on past history, image, reputation, etc.) and the way these may impact on what they hear, the use of language, and so on.

Verbal communication is not only concerned with what individuals say but the way in which they convey their message. Factors may include quality of voice, choice of words and pace of speech. Non-verbal communication will also play a particular role in terms of how the message is conveyed. Examples include posture, eye contact, facial expression and gesticulation. It is argued that the non-verbal messages that we convey frequently demonstrate our true feelings and can be easily detected by colleagues (Gopee & Galloway, 2009). Written communication, such as email, text (SMS) messaging, faxes, hand-written letters and word-processed documents are another commonly used form of communication.

ACTIVITY 3.7

Identify potential limitations of the various types of communication: verbal, non-verbal and written.

Enhancing the clarity of communication

There is great potential for confusion between what the 'sender' of a message wishes to convey and what the 'receiver' hears and understands. Issues such as the emotional state of the people involved, past experiences, perceptions, interruptions, time available and interpretation of non-verbal cues will all impact on the 'receiver's' understanding of the message (Gopee & Galloway, 2009). You may have identified some of these points when working on *Activity 3.6*.

Poor communication can lead to conflict within an organisation (Yoder-Wise, 2003) and can therefore be detrimental to any leadership situation. It is essential that a leader can adapt their style of communication according to the context within which they are operating (Barr & Dowding, 2008).

Weightman (1999) proposes a model of communication, along with a list of check points, to enhance clarity of communication between individuals. It begins with 'encoding' where the 'sender' formulates the message, taking into account the sender's objectives, the nature of the individuals involved in the communication exchange, appropriate use of language and the potential emotional impact of the message. Next, in 'transmitting' the message, the 'sender' considers and uses the best method of communicating the message, ensuring that verbal and non-verbal communication is consistent, use of language is appropriate and that a maximum of seven ideas are transmitted. The 'environment' is also considered in terms of avoidance of interruptions, position and type of seating and coping with distractions. Next, in determining how the message is received ('receiving'), active listening is used to check for understanding of the message. Then, 'decoding' on the part of the 'receiver' takes place and understanding in terms of their ability to make sense of the message, attach any meanings and respond to it needs to be ascertained, again through meaningful dialogue. Finally the 'receiver' provides feedback by encoding their response and conveying their message. This model is applicable to all individual and group interactions and is useful in allowing for identification of potential problems in communication, so that these can be avoided (Barr & Dowding, 2008).

ACTIVITY 3.8

Apply Weightman's model of communication to a leadership situation of your own, where you wish to convey a message, verify understanding and obtain feedback.

Active listening

In applying Weightman's model in *Activity 3.8* you will have addressed active listening. It is therefore useful at this stage to remind ourselves what this entails.

Active listening aims to enhance mutual understanding. It is a method of listening and responding to another person through carefully listening to the message and then repeating it in the speaker's own words to check for understanding. Active listening also involves the use of non-verbal communication such as eye contact, posture and gesture to demonstrate that the listener is paying attention to the speaker's message (Barr & Dowding, 2008). These techniques are denoted by the mnemonic SOLER:

- **S**quarely face the person

- **O**pen your posture

- **L**ean towards the sender

- **E**ye contact maintained

- **R**elax while attending.

Transactional analysis

Transactional analysis is used in leadership to help make sense of both how people interact with each other and also how we treat ourselves (Northouse, 2010). It is based on the work of Eric Berne (1964) which focused on how individuals interact with one another, and how the 'ego states' and certain 'parental drivers' affect each set of interactions or 'transactions'. Transactional analysis asserts that there are three ego states that people use and move in and out of:

- **The Parent:** in this state people unconsciously imitate the behaviour of their parents or parental figures. This state may be nurturing or critical.

- **The Adult:** this state is described as the rational, thinking part of self.

- **The Child:** the state in which people behave, feel and think similarly to how they did in childhood. It can be natural or free or it can be adapted and manipulative, as a survival mechanism.

SCENARIO 3.2

Consider the following examples and identify how the situations outlined may influence which ego state(s) you shift into. Explain your responses.

Conflict

Your manager is angry with you because you took on an additional role without telling him. He shouts at you and tells you that you have lost his trust.

Dynamics

Three people in your team are consistently nasty about Julie, another member of the team. As a result Julie is isolated. You are not sure how to behave; you feel sorry for Julie but you are afraid that you will receive the same treatment from the other three if you challenge them.

Challenge

You are on a night shift and you are the most senior member of staff on duty. A crisis occurs and you have to take charge.

Your responses will be influenced by past experiences and learnt behaviours. Through being aware of how different situations are likely to affect you, you will be able to modify your response as appropriate to the needs of the situation. Responses to conflict and conflict management are addressed in *Chapter 6*.

Berne (1964) outlines 'parental drivers' which could also be argued to be 'societal drivers'. The assertion is that many of us grow up believing that we can stay 'OK' if we obey the following commands:

1. Be perfect
2. Be strong
3. Try hard
4. Please (people)
5. Hurry up.

ACTIVITY 3.9

Consider how these drivers relate to your working life today. To what extent do you still obey these 'commands' and what impact does this have on you and your team?

The *Hurry Up* command may result in people being very efficient as they are motivated to do things in the shortest possible time. However, mistakes can happen due to a lack of preparation. *Be Perfect* is the opposite of *Hurry Up's* style; the individual will want to do things precisely and right the first time. Whilst this is praiseworthy, the risk is that jobs may not be completed on time due to a misjudgement of the time and detail required. Those who try to *Be Strong* are generally able to handle tasks with a sense of calm and can juggle many tasks with skill, but they may not want to show or admit a weakness which may be detrimental to their wellbeing. The *Please People* command results in individuals wanting to please others without people having to ask. They value harmony and make good team members. As a result, however, the individual may be reluctant to challenge others' ideas and may appear passive. The *Try Hard* style is focused on enthusiastically putting effort into a task, and is less concerned about succeeding. The risk associated with this, however, is that the individual may volunteer for more tasks before completing current ones.

By being aware of which drivers may influence us as leaders, we are better able to modify our behaviour to ensure that we work effectively and in the interests of both ourselves and other members of the team.

ASSERTIVENESS

ACTIVITY 3.10

What does the term 'assertiveness' mean to you? Why is it relevant to leadership?

Assertiveness is concerned with *'expressing opinions or desires strongly and with confidence so that people take notice'* (as defined in the Oxford Advanced Learner's Dictionary). In practical terms this may involve behaviours such as:

- Expressing disagreement

- Providing constructive criticism

- Expressing opinions

- Saying no to others

- Allowing others to express their opinions

- Making requests to others

- Making suggestions to others (McCabe & Timmins, 2006; Timmins & McCabe, 2005).

Much of the work underpinning assertiveness is anecdotal. However, it is largely recognised that communication ranges in style, as outlined in *Figure 3.3*:

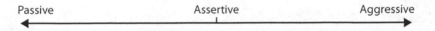

Figure 3.3 *The range of styles in communication*

ACTIVITY 3.11

Study *Figure 3.3*. Outline what the different labels mean and how the styles of communication would be exhibited in terms of behaviour, non-verbal communication and language.

The style in which we communicate will be influenced by the way we perceive ourselves in different contexts, learnt behaviour and personality as well as by the communication skills that we have developed.

Passive behaviour is characterised by the individual not expressing their needs; it is self-devaluing and the individual will generally wait to be led. Non-verbal characteristics include a shrinking posture, a quiet, hesitant voice and little eye contact. Language will be apologetic; for example, *'Sorry to bother you ...'*, or *'It's only my opinion'*. Aggressive communication is characterised by a domineering style where the individual does not listen and focuses on win/lose outcomes. Non-verbal behaviour includes interrupting, staring and pointing. Language is dismissive, allocates blame and may involve shouting. In contrast to the passive and aggressive approaches, assertive behaviour is honest, open and direct, which is reflected in the language used, such as '*I believe /I need /I would like*' and, when appropriate, '*no*'. It recognises the rights of both parties and takes account of what others are voicing. Non-verbal behaviour includes an upright, balanced stance, a firm, clear voice and steady eye contact.

Common barriers to being assertive are the learnt patterns that Berne (1964) outlines, such as not wanting to upset others and acquiescing, as well as concerns regarding others' attitudes towards us. Other issues are a lack of self-belief and a lack of clear intentions.

Practical tips for the development of assertiveness skills include the use of potential scripts such as:

> '*When you* …
>
> *I feel...*
>
> *because...*
>
> *and I would like/need* ...'

SCENARIO 3.3

Diane is consistently late for her span of duty. This causes an inequitable workload for the rest of the team. Diane never acknowledges that she is late or apologises to her colleagues.

Apply the potential script outlined above to this situation. How is Diane likely to react? How will you respond?

Additional tips for developing assertiveness skills include:

- Ensuring that your facts are accurate and that you have them readily available

- Anticipating how others may react to you and preparing your response

- Preparing and using open questions

- Controlling your breathing if you become nervous, by slowing it down and breathing deeply and smoothly.

EMOTIONAL INTELLIGENCE AS A LEADERSHIP TOOL

One of the most significant changes in the leadership literature over recent years has been the recognition that emotional intelligence significantly impacts on leadership performance, with several authors asserting that the most successful leaders are those who have high levels of emotional intelligence (Wall, 2007; Wong & Law, 2002; Goleman, 1998b).

ACTIVITY 3.12

Outline what 'emotional intelligence' means to you.

Emotional intelligence is concerned with the individual's ability to perceive, understand and express emotion. It relates to the individual's ability to both identify their own and others' emotions and to regulate and modify their mood (Goleman, 1995). In relation to leadership, Goleman (1998b) found in an analysis of 'outstanding leaders' that emotional competencies, as opposed to technical and cognitive abilities, accounted for 80–100% of those listed by companies as central to the individual's success. Such competencies included personal competencies such as achievement, self-confidence and commitment as well as social competencies such as influence, political awareness and empathy.

In relation to nursing, Cummings *et al.* (2005) demonstrated that emotionally intelligent nursing leadership can inspire others through channelling emotions, passion and motivation towards the achievement of goals. Such leaders use emotions to mobilise teams, when coaching and in providing the team with a vision for change (Cummings *et al.*, 2005; Watson, 2004). These findings can, arguably, be applied to other areas of health and social care.

Weisinger (2000) asserts that developing self-awareness is vital to the development of emotional intelligence. This is because it is closely related to being able to access one's own resources, the management of emotions, self-motivation, creativity and performance (Akerjordet & Severinsson, 2004; Weisinger, 2000). Weisinger (2000) argues that self-awareness can be enhanced through reflection and exploration of our reactions to people and events. He outlines five 'self-awareness components':

• Examine how you appraise situations

• Make a conscious effort to get in touch with your senses

• Get in touch with your feelings

• Identify what your intentions are

• Be aware of your actions.

More specifically, Vitello-Cicciu (2001) promotes the following questions as a way of focusing on the self:

• What are you feeling now?

• How did you assess this emotion? What verbal and non-verbal cues did you utilise?

- What kind of energy level does this emotion lead to?

- What should you do whilst feeling this way?

- What could happen if the emotion persists?

- What circumstances led to you feeling this way?

- What can you learn from experiencing this emotion?

The Johari window (Luft, 1969), as shown in *Figure 3.4*, is a model that can also be of use in developing self-awareness. It explores four aspects of ourselves: the open area, the blind area, the hidden and the unknown. The open area is the area that we know about ourselves and that others also know about us. Examples may be physical characteristics and personality traits. The blind area is made up of characteristics that others know about us, but we are not aware of. This may include communication skills that others are aware of, but we have no insight into. This area can decrease in size as self-awareness increases through, for example, asking others how we come across in different situations. The hidden area is made up of things that we know about ourselves that we wish to keep private. The 'unknown' is unknown to both ourselves and others. With life experience, this area of the window can become smaller; for example, many new mothers describe surprise at the extreme emotions they feel in relation to their children, that they had previously considered themselves incapable of and that others considered them incapable of too.

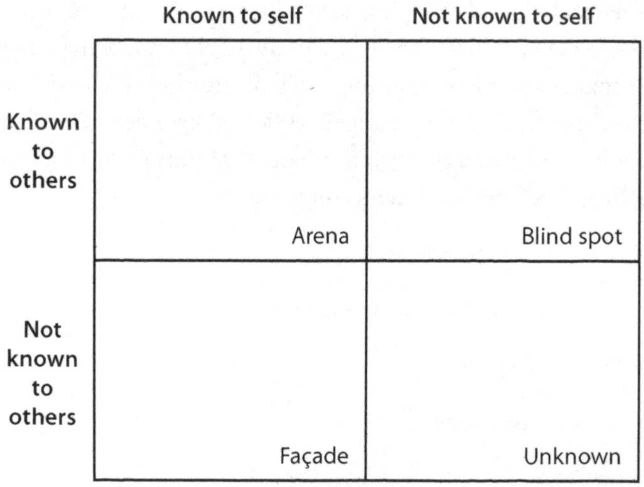

	Known to self	Not known to self
Known to others		
	Arena	Blind spot
Not known to others		
	Façade	Unknown

Figure 3.4 *The Johari window (Luft, 1969)*

ACTIVITY 3.13

Draw out your own Johari window (see *Figure 3.4*) and use it to describe yourself. Team up with a critical friend whose opinion you value to help you decrease the size of your 'blind' area. Adjectives that you may wish to use include:

flexible	organised	adaptable	democratic
assertive	calm	caring	trustworthy
autocratic	tense	confident	dependable
giving	energetic	helpful	charismatic
independent	warm	intelligent	decisive
dominant	knowledgeable	nervous	sympathetic

Additional tools that can aid in this process include maintaining a reflective journal, gauging others' moods based only on sensory feedback and being attentive to our reflex thoughts, intentions and behaviours. The 'NHS 360° Feedback Tool' may also be of use in developing self-awareness and hence emotional intelligence, since it provides an insight into how others perceive our behaviours (NHS Institute for Innovation and Improvement, 2009). Coaching has also been found to be of use in developing emotional intelligence (Wall, 2007); this will be addressed in *Chapter 8*.

CHAPTER SUMMARY

Three key points to take away from Chapter 3:

- A great deal of research has been carried out in identifying skills and qualities that are pivotal in successful leadership, but no definitive list exists because varying qualities and skills will be required by differing contexts. However, the core clusters outlined by the NHS Leadership Qualities Framework provide an evidence-based guide that is pertinent to health and social care.

- Transactional analysis can be of particular use in understanding both inter- and intrapersonal communication.

- Emotional intelligence is a key quality in effective leadership. Its development requires a conscious process that can be enhanced by feedback from others and reflective practice.

QUESTIONS

Question 3.1

Are some people born to lead and some to be led? Explain your answer. *(Learning outcome 3.1)*

Question 3.2

Identify the five skills of an effective leader that you consider to be of most importance. Justify your response. *(Learning outcome 3.2)*

Question 3.3

Review the NHS Leadership Qualities Framework. Which of these qualities do you already possess and which do you need to develop? *(Learning outcome 3.3)*

Question 3.4

List three aspects of your communication skills that you could improve. Outline how you would do this. *(Learning outcome 3.4)*

Question 3.5

What does 'emotional intelligence' mean to you? What would you expect to see in an emotionally intelligent leader? *(Learning outcome 3.5)*

FURTHER READING

Buzan, T. & Buzan, B. (2006) *The Mind Map Book*. Essex: BBC Active for Pearson Education Group.

Goffee, R. & Jones, G. (2000) 'Why should anyone be led by you?' *Harvard Business Review*, **78(5):** 62–70.

Mumford, M.D., Zaccaro, S.J., Harding, F.D., Jacobs, T.O. & Fleishman, E.A. (2000) 'Leadership skills for a changing world: solving complex social problems'. *Leadership Quarterly*, **11(1):** 11–35.

4

LEADERSHIP, VALUES AND CULTURE

LEARNING OUTCOMES:

When you have completed this chapter you should be able to:

4.1 Outline what is meant by culture

4.2 Recognise how values and beliefs link to organisational culture

4.3 Discuss the importance of alignment between personal and organisational objectives

4.4 Understand the relevance of values and culture to leadership.

INTRODUCTION

Having considered what we mean by leadership, the theory which underpins it and the skills and qualities that make for an effective leader, this chapter moves you on to think about the place in which you work and the people you are working with. This can be influenced by whether it is a single organisation (e.g. a private care home), local organisation with many parts, such as a local authority, or one part of a much larger organisation, such as the NHS.

WHAT DO WE MEAN BY CULTURE?

There are many different definitions of organisational culture, which reflects the diversity of organisations in existence. A definition which works well for health and social care is 'the collection of traditions, values, policies, beliefs and attitudes that constitute a pervasive context for everything we do and think in an organisation' (Mullens, 2005 in Barr & Dowding, 2008, p. 174). Another definition is that of Hofstede (2001), who identifies culture as 'the collective programming of the mind that distinguishes the members of one organisation from another'. However, Dowling (1993) has a much simpler way of defining what culture is; he defines it as the '"glue" which holds many organisations together'. Informally, organisational culture is not uncommonly said to be '*the way we do things around here*'.

ACTIVITY 4.1

In relation to the organisation you work in currently, or have worked in previously, what are the things that you would consider make up its 'glue'?

Culture can be thought about not just in terms of the organisation itself but also in relation to the nature of the health and social care area in which you work, such as the community or in an acute hospital, and the different professional groupings with which you work. Barr and Dowding (2008) identify that cultures are affected by:

• the past

• the climate of the present

• the involved technology

• the type of work

• the aims

• the kind of people who work there.

ACTIVITY 4.2

Looking at the list of bullet points above, is there anything else you would now add to your answer to *Activity 4.1*?

Although organisational culture may seem hard to put your finger on, it makes itself visible in a number of different ways to both those working within the organisation and those looking at the organisation from the outside. Hofstede and Hofstede (2005) use the terms 'symbols', 'heroes', 'rituals', 'values' and 'practices' in their model of organisational culture (*Figure 4.1*).

Symbols are the words or visual images that are meaningful for the organisation. This could include the language or phrases used verbally or in internal or external documents, the organisation or departmental logos, the dress code or specialist equipment used, e.g. stethoscopes.

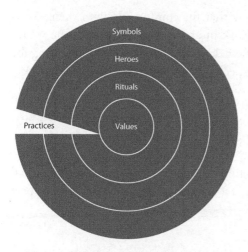

Figure 4.1 *The 'Onion' as a model of organisational culture, adapted from Hofstede (Hofstede & Hofstede, 2005)*

Heroes are the people who are, or have been, associated with the organisation who are admired and are seen as role models for employees or a particular profession because of their expertise, leadership, personality, values or behaviours.

Rituals are activities which take place within the organisation which may or may not be essential but are bound into the organisation. Examples could include informal get-togethers, leaving parties, award ceremonies, etc.

Values are the ideas and beliefs that we hold as special; the things that really matter to us which influence the way we behave and act. They are often said to be innate and are particularly important in the health and social care arena. Many of the health and care professions have particular value sets and philosophical bases which underpin the way they work. These are learnt while they are training in the workplace or studying at college or university.

Practices are the final part of Hofstede's model of organisational culture. This is the slice through the onion that shows the three outer layers and equates to how an outsider sees the culture of an organisation working. However, although the symbols, heroes and rituals are visible to all, it is only by being part of the organisation that they have full meaning and significance.

Hofstede and Hofstede (2005) compare their model to an onion with different layers, with the outermost being the most easy to peel off or change, and values at the core being the hardest to get to and affect. This is because values are something that we learn early on in our lives, at home and in school or college as we grow up. They are influenced by what we see and hear around us and by the time we get into the workplace most of our values are already formed. Normally people tend to behave in a way that fits comfortably with their values and so they usually enter a career, or apply to work in an organisation, where the values align closely with their personal values. Within the field of health and social care, caring for others could be said to be a value, as would be respect for an individual's personal dignity.

From a wider perspective, organisational values usually represent those things that the organisation really believes in. They guide the organisation and its employees towards its goals and they usually relate directly to the purpose for which the organisation exists. Human resource recruitment processes are often designed to ensure that the values of a successful applicant match those of the organisation. In addition to existing at individual and organisational levels, values are often considered at team or departmental level as part of staff development activities.

ACTIVITY 4.3

Reflect on a team that you work in and write a list of the values which you believe that team demonstrates.

Words you thought of might have included some of the following:

- commitment to team goals
- mutual trust and respect
- helpfulness towards one another.

The value terms mentioned above reflect a team where the members are working well together. It would be interesting to ask the other people who you work with what words they would use. The best teamwork happens when there is alignment between the values of the different team members, because this creates a positive climate in which to work, which is why they are often included in team 'away days' or staff development activities. If the different team members do not have similar values it can create conflict and tension, which means the team is less likely to be working effectively. This can also be seen at organisation level. If an individual's personal or professional values do not align with those of the organisation then the working relationship will not be as effective as it might be and could become a source of conflict.

Although many teams in health and social care are multidisciplinary, the individual professions seen, for example, working in the NHS or local authorities such as midwives, allied health professionals, social workers, pharmacists, clinical scientists, project workers, etc. will each have their own cultural identity. As such they are often described as being a subculture with their own symbols, rituals, heroes and values particular to their professional identity. A subculture may be defined as 'a subset of an organisation's members who interact regularly with one another and identify themselves as a distinct group within the organisation, share a set of problems commonly defined to be the problems of all, and routinely take action on the basis of collective understandings unique to the group' (Van Maanen & Barley, in Frost *et al.*, 1985). However, it should be recognised that health and social care professionals will have two sets of values; their professional values and their personal values, both of which can impact on the teams and organisation within which they are working.

ACTIVITY 4.4

Make a list of the different professions that you have worked with recently. What differences or similarities do you see between them in relation to the cultural factors mentioned above? Were there any challenges created by the different cultural identities?

It is not uncommon for some subcultural groups to have difficulty working together or conflict with one another because of the differences in their cultural identity, particularly their values and professional philosophies. Within health and social care settings this is sometimes referred to as 'tribalism' and can be seen as a threat to full inter-professional or interagency working. However, an awareness of these subcultural issues by both team leaders and members of any multidisciplinary team can reduce their impact and in many instances, recognising these differences can strengthen rather than weaken the way that a team works, adding cultural richness.

ETHICS

One particular value which has come more to the fore in recent years is ethical behaviour and organisations often have this overtly within their vision or mission statement.

ACTIVITY 4.5

Think about an organisation or company which identifies itself as having ethical leadership or an ethical approach to its product. Consider why it might use that term and what benefits use of that term might bring to the organisation?

The ability to put yourself forward as an ethical company is seen as a positive thing to do, because it reinforces cultural characteristics that are perceived as important to the public.

This is particularly the case within health and social care organisations where integrity, truth and respect aligned to informed decision-making and confidentiality are perceived as essential ways of working and necessary values within their culture.

French and Bell (1990) modelled their perception of organisational culture on an iceberg floating on the sea, with formal aspects of the organisation visible (above the sea) and the informal aspects invisible (below the surface). This approach confirms still further why culture is seen as a mix of tangible and intangible elements.

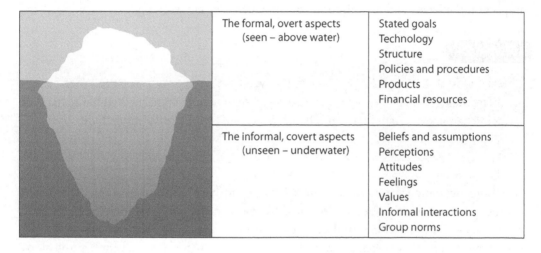

	The formal, overt aspects (seen – above water)	Stated goals Technology Structure Policies and procedures Products Financial resources
	The informal, covert aspects (unseen – underwater)	Beliefs and assumptions Perceptions Attitudes Feelings Values Informal interactions Group norms

Figure 4.2 *The 'Iceberg' model of organisational culture (adapted from French & Bell, 1990)*

A further model of organisational culture which helps to demonstrate the complexity of organisational culture, and how one element influences another, is Johnson and Scholes' cultural web (2005). This is an expansion of the Hofstedes' work which adds routines, stories, power structures, control systems and the organisational structure itself (*Figure 4.3*).

Routines are placed along with rituals as they reinforce the activities that take place within the organisation, particularly those which happen on a day-to-day or weekly basis, such as case conferences, ward rounds, team meetings, etc.

Stories are the way that members of an organisation share successes, failures, near misses and important events with one another and those outside the organisation, which reinforce what is perceived as being important to the organisation.

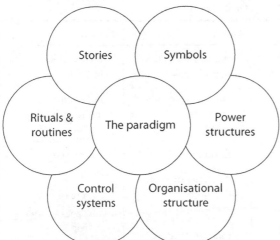

Figure 4.3 *The cultural web (adapted from Johnson and Scholes (2005))*

Power structures relate to where the sources of power sit within the organisation (see also *Chapter 5*). It is individuals or groups of people who hold the power to shape core values and beliefs and, therefore, influence organisational culture. Particular values can be encouraged or discouraged through workplace systems, e.g. appraisal or performance reviews.

Control systems place emphasis on what matters to the organisation, such as the achievement of targets, successful inspections and effective budgeting. Systems that measure outcomes can influence individual behaviour, particularly if they are linked in any way to reward.

Organisational structure reflects the roles and relationships and power systems that promote a particular culture. A hierarchical structure will produce a culture that is very different from that of a flat organisation where there are very few levels or grades between the highest and the lowest employees.

At the centre of the web is the paradigm, i.e. the assumptions that exist within the organisation. Johnson and Scholes (2005) identified that it is these assumptions that are often the most intangible and, therefore, difficult to identify and explain within an organisation.

Handy (1985) identified four different types of organisational culture, as outlined in *Table 4.1*.

Table 4.1 *Handy's four types of organisational culture (Handy, 1985)*

Role	Task	Power	Person
– based around job – hierarchical structure – predictable and stable – inflexible – rigid – barriers between different departments – impersonal – suppresses individuality – change is slow, brought about by fear	– central figure for strength – communication radiates from the centre – dominance from the centre – responds to change quickly – small organisations – politics important, knowing what the boss wants – can exert strict internal control – conform or GO	– successful solution to problems – performance judged by results and problems solved – flexible – decisions made at junctions – more loosely bound than role culture – power influenced from various positions – respect and power from individual knowledge	– focuses solely on the individual – not common for the entire organisation – usually in small areas of large companies – culture of educated articulate individuals – specialist with common interests, e.g. researcher – operates independently

ACTIVITY 4.6

Make a list of different parts of your organisation and identify which type of organisational culture identified by Handy they are most like.

Handy's model of types of organisational cultures is useful when looking at both large and small organisations. For example, Barr and Dowding (2008) perceive that the NHS as a whole can be seen as a role culture, with small project teams within it working in a task culture. They suggest that research teams, high-dependency care and operating theatres are good examples where there is a power culture. Person culture exists to a lesser extent; however, it could be conceived where there is a very small department of just one person, for example a specialist practitioner. A similar diversity of cultures can also be seen within local authorities and independent or voluntary sector providers.

An alternative approach is put forward by Kanter (1983), who suggests that there are just two types of culture: segmentalist and integrative, as identified in *Table 4.2*.

Table 4.2 *Segmentalist and integrative culture (Kanter, 1983)*

Segmentalist culture
• views organisational problems narrowly
• locates problems and hence responsibilities narrowly within department's or individual's remit
• has segmented structure divided into departments and functions, often working against one another
• shuns experimentation
• avoids confronting problems and conflicts
• has weak coordinating mechanisms
• emphasises precedent, policies, procedures and systems
• is inward looking
Integrative culture
• sees problems as related
• views problems and responsibilities as shared and connected
• has matrix or team/project-based structure
• innovates and tests, inviting experimentation
• creates mechanisms of coordination for sharing information and ideas
• looks for novel solutions
• is outward looking

The two lists of characteristics Kanter identifies are opposites in many instances and it must be recognised that few organisations will sit completely under either heading.

ACTIVITY 4.7

Do you work in a mainly segmentalist or integrative culture? Can you list the reasons why you believe this?

The particular value of Kanter's two-type model can be seen in relation to change. She believes that organisations which have all or many of the integrative features are more likely to be able to cope with change or even thrive in a dynamic environment. She argues that segmentalist cultures are much slower to respond and can struggle when required to change.

ACTIVITY 4.8

Does Kanter's opinion regarding the ability to respond to change match your perception of your organisation's culture identified in *Activity 4.6*?

CULTURAL IDENTITY BEYOND THE ORGANISATION

It is important to remember, however, that health and social care organisations seldom exist in isolation. There is often a local, regional or national organisational perspective which needs to be taken into consideration. Even if, for example, a care home or community project is a 'one-off' it will usually be linked into a network of organisations in one way or another.

The NHS is a prime example of a big national organisation which is influenced by the cultural identity of the United Kingdom. Brooks (2009) identifies what he considers to be the elements which impact on the society in which we grow up and work and so influence how values develop and lead to a national culture.

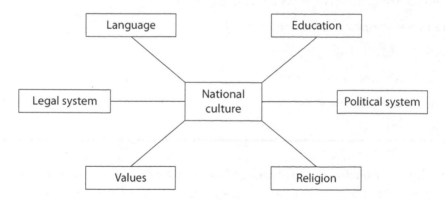

Figure 4.4 *Factors affecting national culture, adapted from Brooks (2009)*

However, although there is an over-arching organisational national culture, there are four regional subcultures relating to the four countries which make up the UK. This is apparent within the NHS; the way the NHS is structured and managed is very different in those four countries, as can be seen in *Chapter 7*. In addition, there are further differences, because each of those large regions is broken down into smaller parts. For example, in England there are a number of Strategic Health Authorities (SHAs) which demonstrate slightly different approaches to health care. Their approaches are dependent upon local factors such as population size, demography and geographical factors as well as the influence of the people employed within the SHAs themselves. It is, therefore, understandable that when organisations or structures separate out or merge, there are often tensions or sources of conflict as the different cultures 'collide'. This can particularly be seen where organisations which have significant cultural differences merge or have to work more closely together, such as the new combined community and acute NHS trusts. This is why the management of change (see *Chapter 6*) will often include attention to cultural issues, and an understanding of culture is vital in those leading the change processes.

WORKING BEYOND THE NATIONAL CULTURE?

A considerable amount of investigation and analysis has taken place in relation to the differences between the national cultures of different countries. Hofstede (1980, 1984, 1991) is seen as a major writer in this area and his model of four cultural dimensions is easy to use and understand. He collected a large amount of data on the attitudes of employees from 50 countries. These dimensions are referred to as power distance, individualism, uncertainty avoidance and masculinity/femininity.

Power distance is the social distance between people of different rank or position. In some countries subordinates are less likely to question the decisions or actions of their managers. In other countries it is the norm for subordinates to debate issues with their superiors and be part of the decision-making process.

Individualism relates to the extent to which an individual relies on a group approach (collectivism) to solving problems and making decisions or is more likely to take individual initiative.

Uncertainty avoidance reflects the attitudes towards ambiguity. Some cultures have a high level of avoidance whereas others have a low uncertainty avoidance.

Masculinity/femininity is a complex variable which reflects values that are widely perceived to be more masculine, such as assertiveness, competitiveness and results orientation. Femininity on the other hand is seen to be more cooperative and to show greater awareness of feelings and equal opportunities.

The awareness of the above factors relating to different countries' national cultural identities is important in the world today as the global workforce is more mobile. In the UK the health and social care workforce is drawn from a multinational pool and an understanding of the different cultural dimensions is invaluable to leaders at all levels within the organisation, as these differences can either be a source of confusion leading to tension or add richness within the workplace.

CULTURAL GAP

There can also be a gap between the kind of culture that an organisation currently has and that which its senior management would like it to have. This is called a cultural gap, and much time is often spent trying to understand what constitutes this gap so that the organisation can work towards closing it in order to create a stronger organisational culture. This in turn is more likely to lead to organisational success. Having a shared commitment to organisational goals and values increases levels of motivation, creates stability and encourages teamwork. It also facilitates good decision-making and more effective working (Deal & Kennedy, 1982). It should be noted that an organisation may also use the recruitment process to employ new staff who 'fit' the profile they aspire to, as well as working on closing the cultural gap.

SO WHY IS UNDERSTANDING OF CULTURE IMPORTANT IN LEADERSHIP?

Although organisational culture is created by a number of different factors within the organisation, it is important to remember that culture is dynamic and constantly evolving. Although it is recognised that it is difficult to change culture, it is possible to do so under the right leadership. However, you have to be able to recognise the existing culture before you can do anything about it and you need to be aware of the culture you want to move to (Brooks and Bate, 1994).

ACTIVITY 4.9

Choose an element of culture in your workplace that you would like to change in some way. This could be a negative feature that you want to stop or a positive one that you want to enhance further. What could you do or say differently that might have an impact?

Through recognising what the keystones of culture are, you can begin to influence the team, department or organisational culture through reinforcing positive behaviours, discouraging less welcome behaviours or through considering your own words, actions and the symbols that you use; you can shape the practices that others see. A knowledge of culture can enable you to better understand how your organisation works, or doesn't work, or recognise when and how it is trying to change. Knowledge of culture can also help you improve your understanding of your own personal and professional values and enable you to gain an insight into your personal needs and motivations and reflect on why you appear to 'fit' well into a particular organisation or work context. One of the challenges of leadership can be ensuring that the decisions and actions that you take reflect and align with both your personal values and the values of the organisation.

Schein (1985) identified that there was a relationship between leadership and cultural formation within his model of organisational culture. He believed that leadership needed to be seen in context and in the culture of that context, as illustrated in *Table 4.3*. He suggested that there were two continuums, and that neither one was better than the other; they were just different.

Table 4.3 *Schein's relationship between leadership and culture formation (Schein, 1985)*

– operate independently	– ideas valued from older, wiser and higher status individuals
– ideas valued from any individual	
– people are responsible, motivated and capable of governing themselves	– people are capable of loyalty and discipline in carrying out directions
– conflict is OK and can be sorted out through groups	– relationships are lineal and vertical
	– each individual has a place in the organisation
– group members will care for each other	– the organisation is responsible for taking care of its members

As you can see, your actions and words as a leader will make a difference to the culture within your workplace and it is suggested that there is a correlation between a strong positive culture and organisational performance (Deal & Kennedy, 1982). It is usually the culture that a leader tries to change in order to improve the quality of the services being delivered and in achieving objectives. Most organisations welcome employee participation in strengthening the organisation and this is particularly the case within health and social care as this usually has a positive impact on the service user and carer experience. With a knowledge and understanding of culture you will put yourself in an excellent position to actively participate in such activities and so be able to raise your profile as a potential leader at team, departmental, organisational or even national level.

CHAPTER SUMMARY

Three key points to take away from Chapter 4:

- Different types of organisational culture exist and affect the sort of team you work in. It can be tangible or intangible, visible or unseen, and different models exist which can help you analyse how culture is expressed within an organisation.

- Knowledge and understanding of culture can help you as a leader; they enable you to influence it and so potentially improve team performance and/or the service user experience.

- The alignment of personal and organisational values is important in enabling a strong culture to support organisational success.

QUESTIONS

Question 4.1

Outline what you understand to be the meaning of culture. *(Learning outcome 4.1)*

Question 4.2

Using your own workplace as an example, identify how the values of your organisation reflect its culture. *(Learning outcome 4.2)*

Question 4.3

Discuss why it is important that personal and organisational values and objects are aligned. *(Learning outcome 4.3)*

Question 4.4

Outline why you believe that an understanding of the relevance of values and culture is important to a leader. *(Learning outcome 4.4)*

FURTHER READING

Barr, J. & Dowding, L. (2008) *Leadership in Healthcare*. London: Sage.

Brooks, I. (2009) *Organisational Behaviour: Individuals, Groups and Organisation*, 4th edition. Harlow: Pearson.

5

LEADERSHIP, POWER AND INFLUENCE

LEARNING OUTCOMES:

When you have completed this chapter you should be able to:

5.1 Outline the different bases and sources of power and how they can be interrelated

5.2 Understand the significance of words, deeds and symbols

5.3 Describe ways in which you can influence outcomes

5.4 Recognise how and where leadership can take place.

INTRODUCTION

In previous chapters we looked at the skills and qualities that leaders can use in order to lead effectively. We also identified that different forms of leadership occur depending on the situation, context and culture of the workplace. In this chapter you will begin to consider what 'power' is and where that power comes from – its source or base – and how you can influence what happens in the workplace. You will also start to think about the impact of politics, both within your organisation or externally, locally or nationally and how they affect the way you work.

SO WHAT IS POWER?

ACTIVITY 5.1

Consider a situation in either your personal life or at work where someone exerted power over you. What made you feel you should do what they wanted you to do? Why did you feel that they were more powerful than you and that you should do as they asked?

One definition of power is 'the potential ability to influence behaviour, to change the course of events, to overcome resistance, and to convince people to do things that they would not do otherwise' (Pfeffer, 1992, p. 30) or to put it more simply, the ability to make things happen. However, there are underlying reasons why someone can 'make things happen'.

SOURCES AND BASES OF POWER

The use of source or base of power as a descriptor to identify where power comes from varies from author to author. However, the best-known work in this area is by French and Raven (1959), who identified five main sources of power: reward power, coercive power, expert power, legitimate power and reverent power. Each of these sources is dependent on the attitudes and values, and therefore the perception, of the recipients in order for them to function as sources of power as well as the relationship between those wielding the power and recipients.

Reward power is that which comes from an individual's ability to provide rewards or benefits. This could be in monetary terms – a salary rise or bonus – or perks such as working the shifts you want to or being able to book the annual leave time that you would prefer; however, this sort of power can also be used negatively to withhold those same rewards or benefits.

Coercive power depends on fear and comes from the capacity of an individual or organisation to punish or impose sanctions. This is a very negative type of power and although it usually produces immediate results, it seldom leads to long-term commitment. One example of coercive power is often seen at meetings. One or more people want to say something; however, there can be undercurrent relating to what cannot be said – an 'unwritten' rule of not upsetting the applecart – because of a certain person or persons also being at the table. If the 'forbidden subject' is raised it can lead to individuals being 'punished', for example informally by being given poor off-duty hours or more difficult patients or clients to look after. In some instances it can even lead to reasons being 'found' that exclude the 'troublemaker' from meetings. The individual therefore does or doesn't do something they know they should, because they are scared by the potential consequences if they go against the 'unwritten' rules.

The health and social care sector is highly regulated and inspected, and as such you may 'feel' as though this type of power is more present than in other sectors. There are targets to be met, procedures and processes to follow that are organisationally critical; however, unless people believe in what they are doing and why, coercive power may be used to ensure compliance, which has only short-term impact, rather than lead to a long-term change in practice.

Expert power is based on the perception that an individual or organisation has special skills or knowledge. This is particularly the case for those working in health and social care as there are so many different people who could be looking after just a single client or patient – paramedics, care assistants, associate practitioners, social workers, nurses, doctors, allied health professionals, pharmacists, etc. and so many specialist fields of care, e.g. learning disabilities, drug misuse, end of life, older adults or neonates, to name just a few.

Legitimate power relates to the position or role that a person holds within an organisation. That is particularly the case in hierarchical organisations (see *Chapter 4*) or where regulatory or statutory bodies are involved. The care sector in particular can be very hierarchical – both formally through job grading but also informally within multidisciplinary teams (MDT), where one profession is sometimes seen as holding more sway than another in decision-making. However, sometimes it is not the most senior person who holds the power. For example, a consultant may wish to discharge a patient or client; however, it may be that a home visit by an occupational therapist or an assessment by a social worker holds the power to that outcome being achieved (see section on paradox of power, below).

Reverent power relates to the respect in which an individual or an organisation is held. An example of this would be an eminent consultant who is admired for their commitment to work in a particular field over and above that engendered by their expert status, or a care worker whom all the clients and co-workers in a home admire and like, and would do that little bit more for.

Robbins (1984) agreed with French and Raven that someone's expertise or position might be a source of power; however, he considered that the way in which they could exert that power was a different entity. He called these mechanisms of exerting influence bases of power. A manager has power through their position but if they also control resources then they have the ability to influence outcomes through the control of budgets or rewards. Coercive power may relate, in particular, to rules and procedures in health and social care, where the sector is highly regulated and inspections or audits happen on a regular basis. However, as mentioned above, it is also an area where significant expert power is evident. *Table 5.1* illustrates the differences Robbins proposed between sources and bases of power.

Table 5.1 *Robbins' sources and bases of power (Robbins, 1984)*

Sources of power	Bases of power
Coercive power	Control of budgets
Expert power	Control of rewards
Legitimate/position power	Persuasion
Reverent power	Rules and procedures
	Physical presence
	Charisma

As far as Mintzberg (1983) is concerned, the terms power and influence can be used interchangeably. For him there are five major sources of power: control of a resource, control of a skill, control of a critical body of knowledge, legal prerogatives (the rights or privileges to impose choices) and, lastly, access to those who possess the first four sources in this list. He also suggests that it is not enough to have simply a source of power; you also need to expend energy in a politically skilful way in order to influence effectively. Access to resources can be considered in the broadest sense in that they could be financial; however, they could also include access to equipment or access to information or even access to people through a group or committee.

Morgan (1996) identified still further possible sources of power (see *Table 5.2*), although he included areas that other authors might consider bases rather than sources. You can see there is some consistency between all the authors mentioned so far; however, more potential sources or bases have been identified as the subject of power has been considered over the years.

Table 5.2 *Morgan's sources of power (adapted from Morgan, 1996 in Brooks, 2009)*

Role or position authority
Control of limited resources
Use of the structure, rules and regulations of the organisation
Decision-making process control
Control of information
Control of boundaries
Negative capability
Control of technology
Personal networks and links through informal leadership
Management of symbolism
Gender relations and their management
Control of timelines
Level of personal power

Northouse (2010) identifies two major kinds of power in organisations – position power and personal power. His definition of position power is not dissimilar to that identified by French and Raven, in that it relates to the status of an individual within the organisation and includes legitimate power, reward power and coercive power. However, he also identifies personal power, which he defines as the influence that a leader gains from their followers either by being liked, being seen as a good role model or being very skilled in their profession, i.e. reverent power or expert power. These are the two sources of power that any member of an organisation can aspire to as they do not rely on any particular status or position of power. It is this personal power, therefore, which enables leaders to emerge at all levels of an organisation, no matter what their role or profession. This premise is supported by the work of Kotter (1985) who also suggests that influence and leadership are inextricably bound together.

ACTIVITY 5.2

Identify examples of when you have seen the different types of power described above taking place. How did the use of these sources or bases of power impact on the work you were doing?

Within health and social care there has to be a considerable amount of teamwork to deliver the services needed, whether you are working in the community or in an operating theatre. However, these teams are often divided into either professional groupings or client-specific multidisciplinary teams. In addition, there are often a number of different agencies involved, either because a case is complex or because of the setting in which the care is taking place. This means that although you are usually working towards a single goal there can be tensions because of the power differentials held by the different professionals or non-professionals involved.

ACTIVITY 5.3

How many people from different professional or non-professional backgrounds have you come across at work in the past week? Can you identify what their sources or bases of power were? If they were working with you in relation to a single patient or client, would there be any 'pecking' order in relation to the power held by a particular colleague – and if so, why?

A number of people are involved in any health and social care situation or activity, such as in *Activity 5.3*. There is, therefore, the potential for tension and conflict. Brooks (2009) identifies that 'conflict is apparent when at least one party perceives that it exists and where an interest or concern of that party is about to be or has been compromised or frustrated'. Conflict is not uncommon between individuals within a team or a department. Indeed inter-departmental conflict or conflict between different levels within an organisation can create a variety of leadership challenges, depending on the source of the conflict. Pondy (1967, in Barr & Dowding, 2008) identifies a four-stage model of conflict, as outlined in *Table 5.3*.

Table 5.3 *Four-stage model of conflict (Pondy, 1967 in Barr & Dowding, 2008)*

Perceived conflict is where there is a feeling of unease.

Felt conflict is where the conflict is internalised and agreed as a real conflict of interests.

Manifest conflict is where the conflict is externalised and expressed.

Conflict aftermath is where the outcome of the conflict episode affects the individual(s) and group(s) concerned.

ACTIVITY 5.4

Identify an incident you have experienced within the last month when conflict arose. What do you feel was the source of the conflict?

Whilst the cause of conflict may relate to individual differences, it may also be linked to differences in ideology and personal objectives. Barr and Dowding (2008) identify seven potential causes of conflict:

- differences in action at various levels of the organisation
- concealed objectives
- limited resources
- departmentalisation and specialisation
- nature of work processes and design
- role conflict
- inequitable treatment.

Conflict management is addressed in *Chapter 6*.

SCENARIO 5.1

Tom is a project worker for a family living in rented accommodation. The family is on the point of being evicted. The children are on the edge of care and Tom believes that it would be in the family's interests to remain where they are living to enable the Family Intervention Project (FIP) worker to work with the family in a familiar environment. The Housing Association who own the property want to evict the family.

In the situation outlined in *Scenario 5.1*, the Housing Association could have hard evidence to back their decision to be seeking eviction, possibly in the form of rent arrears or antisocial behaviour. Tom might have evidence from previous cases that moving a family at this time will increase rather than decrease the family's issues and that the children are more likely to be taken into care, but it is not 'hard' evidence and, therefore, not as powerful as that of the Housing Association. Therefore, there could be a source of conflict, because resolution is different for the parties involved. However, the Housing Association might wish to appear to be good landlords and offer the family a further opportunity through their commitment to work with the FIP worker, and Tom may be able to use previous evidence (suitably anonymised) to support his case.

Brooks (2009) identifies that there are three further aspects of power that he believes are important: negative power, covert power and powerlessness.

Negative power is influence which is exerted to either resist or disrupt activity. It is particularly seen in organisations when change is being undertaken and, if used effectively, it can slow down or sometimes even prevent activity from happening. An example of this could be seen in relation to the Conservative–Liberal Democrat coalition government plans put forward in the White Paper *Equity and Excellence: Liberating the NHS* (Department of Health, 2010a). Such was the strength of feeling about some of the proposals that the parliamentary process was 'paused' whilst the Future Forum conducted a listening exercise to evaluate the concerns being raised. It could, however, also be said that the 'pause' occurred because of the reverent power and expert power of some of the individuals and groups raising their issues.

Covert power is the term Brooks (2009) uses to identify power which is invisible or transparent. A human resource department can 'slow down' the appointment process, thus making subtle cost savings, or the dissemination of information can be controlled by limiting its circulation, the timing of its release or accelerating or slowing down how it is released. In addition, this type of power can be used to influence what items appear on a meeting agenda or when a meeting is held and who is invited.

ACTIVITY 5.5

Compare and contrast when different meetings are held in your organisation; what time are they held and how long are they? How often are they held? Who is able to put items onto the agenda? Are there direct links to power as identified above?

Another aspect of influence related to meetings is the personal interactions of those present, which can directly affect the outcome of the meeting.

SCENARIO 5.2

Claire is a social worker taking part in a case conference concerning the discharge of an older client with a learning disability. The other members of the multidisciplinary team seem restless and not actively engaged when Claire is speaking. One person is responding by nodding and occasionally saying 'yes'; however, the others are looking past Claire or down at their papers. The meeting does not go the way that Claire was hoping and she feels that she has let the client down.

ACTIVITY 5.6

Think about a recent occasion when you have spoken and tried to influence people. This can be anything such as speaking at a case conference, participating in a ward round or taking part in a workshop. Consider the reactions of the other people present to what you said and write down why you think they reacted as they did.

When trying to influence somebody it is really important that you engage them actively in the conversation or debate. If you prepare well prior to meetings it is likely that when you do start to speak, you won't take too long to get to the point and you will be able to speak clearly because you are less nervous. Making eye contact as you speak is also important, as this actively engages others' attention. You also need to consider the way in which the other person might like to receive information. The reactions that Claire experienced would suggest that she needed to plan differently for the meeting. One way forward would be to approach the professional who did engage with her and ask for their thoughts on how the meeting had gone and if they had any suggestions to offer Claire for future meetings. Influencing is an important skill for a leader so it is very important that you are seen as a good communicator, able to get your point across in a clear way. This skill is discussed and expanded upon in *Chapter 3*.

POWERLESSNESS

Powerlessness is '*a real or perceived state of having little or no power*' (Brooks, 2009, p. 241). Many staff often feel powerless within an organisation, because they perceive they have little control over organisational decisions and are unsupported in their work. However, Brooks differentiates between real powerlessness, where individuals have limited or no sources or bases of power, and perceived powerlessness, which is dependent upon whether an individual actually wants power and their perception of themselves compared to others within the team or organisation. Block (1987) identified that the negative politics and bureaucracy which exist in organisations can make people feel powerless and reduce their energy levels.

However, he believes that if managers can reduce the level of control over decision-making and responsibility then employees have an increased sense of ownership and responsibility. That is, they will feel less powerless and more empowered. Empowerment can be described as a process which enhances feelings of personal ability in individuals through positive personal feedback, as well as the identification and removal of the organisational factors that lead to the feeling of powerlessness. This in turn leads to 'the belief in one's capabilities to organise and execute the courses of action required to manage prospective situations' (Bandura, 1995).

The desire to create an environment in which staff would feel empowered throughout an organisation was one of the main reasons underpinning the development of the Leadership at the Point of Care and NHS Leading an Empowered Organisation (LEO) programmes.

ACTIVITY 5.7

Are you empowered or powerless within your work place? Why do you feel this way? What could you do to increase your sense of empowerment, if appropriate? How could you take the lead to make this happen for others?

It can be argued that empowerment can actually increase the overall amount of power within an organisation, with senior managers actually gaining power because of the increase in morale and productivity gained by devolving a degree of decision-making and autonomy downwards. However, an organisation needs to take great care when empowering staff not to make their leaders and managers feel disempowered, otherwise empowerment can actually lead to overall negative rather than positive results. Also, if empowerment is to make a real difference there must be total organisational commitment, otherwise some areas will 'hoard' knowledge and decision-making responsibility, which will cause the overall process to fail (Lloyd, 1996).

ABUSE OF POWER

Those in power can also abuse that power, though they may not always realise that they are doing so. An example of a situation when this could occur is the hospital ward round where the lead doctor and a number of members of the multidisciplinary team, and also possibly students, gather around a patient's bed to discuss their condition, treatment and progress. It is very easy for this to become a conversation held over the patient rather than including them in the discussions – particularly in a teaching hospital. In addition, the staff are likely to be in uniform and the patient in pyjamas and the staff standing up and therefore high above the level of the patient, who is likely to be in a chair or bed. These are all elements which take power away from the patient, albeit unintentionally. An imbalance, or even abuse, of power can also occur within the same situation amongst members of the team, with certain members assuming greater power than others. If abused, this power can be used to silence colleagues, which may ultimately compromise care.

TRANSFER OF POWER

Sometimes it is essential that power is transferred from one individual to another in a transparent way.

SCENARIO 5.3

Joe is a paramedic attending an elderly person who has fallen at home. Whilst he is taking the patient into hospital, he is in charge of her care; however, shortly after they arrive in A&E he needs to pass that role to the person in charge there, and then A&E will need to pass that role on to a member of a ward team when she is admitted. After Joe arrives at A&E there is a short wait until the A&E team are ready to take responsibility for the elderly woman; however, Joe knows she remains his responsibility in the meantime.

There needs to be a clear transfer of power from Joe to a nurse or doctor in A&E and then a further transfer of power to the ward nurse. This is a good example of 'situational' power, as described in *Chapter 2*. It is vital, however, that the power is retained with one person until it is officially transferred and that there is absolute clarity between the two leaders, i.e. there is a clear demarcation of where responsibility lies, and when it is transferred, to ensure continuity of care.

THE PARADOX OF POWER

No matter how much positional power an individual has, there can be occasions when they are actually powerless; their power is actually, in part, dependent on other people (Lloyd, 1996). This can be because they are not in overall control of everything that impacts on an activity. Alternatively they may not have all the knowledge or the skills required to undertake an action, or there may be multiple stakeholders involved with many different bases and sources of power to contend with. For example, a consultant may not be able to discharge a patient unless a home visit has taken place or care services set up. Calabria (1982) called this the paradox of power.

ACTIVITY 5.8

Consider your line manager. Think of a situation where they would be powerless and then identify why that is the case.

SO WHY IS UNDERSTANDING THE NATURE OF POWER IMPORTANT TO YOU?

Kotter (1985) suggests that influence and leadership are inextricably bound together and, as you have seen above, several bases of power are related to influence rather than position within an organisation. It is, therefore, possible to become a leader at any level within an organisation. If you have, or can develop, the skills and attributes that enable you to influence others within your workplace (or personal life!) then you will be more likely to be able to influence outcomes and begin to unleash your potential as a leader.

IDENTIFYING SOURCES OF INFLUENCE

ACTIVITY 5.9

Review what you have done in your personal or work life over the past week. Was there an occasion when you had to act in a certain way, take a particular approach or choose your words with care in order to change the way something happened? Or did something happen that afterwards you wished you had handled differently? Reflect on what you did – or wished you had done – and relate that to the sources and bases of power identified above.

Figure 5.1 identifies clearly the process by which power can influence outcome.

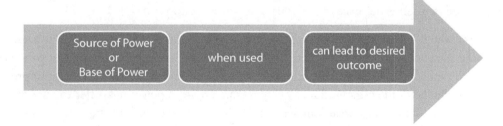

Figure 5.1 *The process of influencing*

By trying to influence an outcome you were using personal power to achieve a result, and as such trying to take the lead in the situation. Owen (2010) suggests several ways in which you can increase your influence, including borrowing the influence from others and becoming a problem solver. If you step in to chair a meeting or lead a team in the absence of the role holder, you inherit some of their credibility by taking on their mantle. If you can propose a way of resolving an issue facing a respected colleague, when resolution occurs and they disseminate what was done, you gain the benefit not just from being recognised as the issue solver but also from the linkage of your name with that of the respected colleague in relation to the solution.

Jayne has been a care assistant for 12 months and can see a way in which the wellbeing of the older people she is working with could improve through enhancing their social activities. The home matron is feeling under pressure to deliver fundamental care relating to hydration and doesn't see enhancing social activities as a priority. Jayne wants to lead a project to improve the situation.

Identify ways in which Jayne could successfully achieve this outcome.

One of the ways in which to gain support is to hold good conversations about current issues with key people who are respected within the organisation. This can be done by asking open questions (a question which cannot be answered by just replying 'yes' or 'no') that have a clear purpose, to encourage them to share their thoughts and feelings. It is also important to keep focused on the conversation, listen carefully to the responses and paraphrase back to the other person what they have said, so that they feel you understand their position. Effective listening will also help to build their trust in you and a rapport between you (see *Chapter 3*). By communicating in this way you get to know more about the person, what really matters to them and what they need – or don't need. You are also gaining information which you can use at a later date to influence them. In addition, when that member of staff or manager has to consider a matter to which you are linked, they should be positively influenced by their experience of previous interactions with you.

Another way to gain influence is to offer to attend a meeting for a colleague who is pressed for time. Not only will you please them by giving them some unexpected space, but you may also gain exposure to different people and a better insight into an unknown area, or improve your knowledge of the organisation. When you are attending meetings, offer to take notes or act as a facilitator for a break-out session or give the report back to the group. This will raise your profile but also it is a way to take control; a facilitator controls the direction of discussions and the reporter or note taker can influence what is summarised from a session. These are often tasks that others find difficult or people are too busy to take on; however, they are an excellent way of gaining influence as well as drawing attention to yourself as a potential leader.

In Jayne's case (*Activity 5.10*) by holding a conversation with her team leader, who was well respected by the matron, about the hydration, she could have gained a better understanding of the issue and the team leader might then have felt an increased rapport with Jayne. Jayne could also have talked to various service users and their carers to gain their trust so that she could build into her proposed activities those which would not only contribute to solving the issue but, in addition, be well received by the people who really mattered – the service users and carers. When she had the opportunity to raise the idea with the matron Jayne could have then used the borrowed power from both her team leader and the service users and carers to demonstrate how her idea could contribute to solving the hydration issue and improving the wellbeing of the service users. Jayne might then have been asked to lead the project.

Being a problem solver is an excellent way to develop into a leader. If you can see a way in which to improve the service being offered to service users or patients and then find the right opportunity to discuss this with the person whose responsibility it is to deliver the service, you can help them achieve their short-term goals. This will help you gain influence not just at that moment in time but in the future – as well as achieve your initial idea of improving the service. Remember, new ideas are not just based on the idea itself but on the perception of the person putting forward the idea.

Personal image can be very important in your pathway to becoming a leader. Dress codes vary tremendously – working on a ward in an acute hospital trust is very different from a community centre; however, there are ways in which you can work out what is appropriate. Dress is a form of non-verbal communication; it says a lot about you before you say a word or complete an action, and you will be judged on how you look (neat, messy, professional, appropriate) and behave (smiling, frowning, hand gestures, a more direct or focused gaze). Therefore you need to consider the impression that you offer to either service users or your colleagues (Gabbott and Hogg, 2001).

SYMBOLS AND WORDS

Pfeffer (1981) identifies that there are five ways of assessing the level of influence of an individual within an organisation:

* Determinants: an individual's access to sources of influence

* Consequences: finding out who benefits (or doesn't benefit) from decisions being made

* Symbols: the trappings of power

* Reputation

* Representation.

You have already learnt about four of these; however, the final one is equally important. The purpose of a symbol is to convey a meaning. A symbol can be a very powerful way of getting a message across to a large number of people without the use of words or explanations. The same symbols can have different meanings in different contexts and for different people; however, the relationship between a symbol and what it represents is often arbitrary.

Several television programmes have been set in hospitals. Make a list of the different symbols you have seen that relate to power. Can you see differences in the symbols between a programme set in the present and one which is set in the past?

Within the health service many symbols are used as badges of power. In the past the seniority of a nurse would be identified by the type of hat she wore; the complexity of the design related directly to her status, i.e. a legitimate power source. Nowadays it is often the colour of the uniform that differentiates different staff grades, or agency staff from permanent staff. When a member of the public sees a person with a stethoscope around their neck, they usually immediately think they are a doctor, despite the fact that many different health professionals use stethoscopes! A white coat or a uniform are accepted as being symbolic of a 'professional'. In reality this is no longer the normal attire in many care settings; however, what people 'see' is not always based on reality but on 'perceived' reality, such as that which they see on the television.

There are other emblems of power which can be seen throughout organisations: the size and location of an office, the presence of a car parking space, whether refreshments are available at a meeting or not. A smartly dressed person amongst others who are less well turned out is often assumed to be a manager or more senior member of staff. A significant amount of energy is often spent on the design of an organisation logo to ensure it projects the desired image, i.e. that it is the right 'kind' of symbol. This can also be the case with, for example, the size of a nameplate on a door, or the title by which someone is known. Consider the doctor who has gained legitimate power through being addressed as Dr X for many years who becomes a consultant – and reverts to being a Mr or Ms!

POLITICS AND POWER

Organisational politics can be defined as 'activities to acquire, develop and use power and other resources to obtain one's preferred outcome when there is uncertainty or disagreements about choices' (Daft, 1983). However, this applies to everyday life as well as organisations! Baron and Greenberg (1990) identified four 'triggers' of political activities: the existence of uncertainty, the scarcity of resources, organisational conflict and where organisational units have equal power. It is, therefore, no surprise that politics exists in and affects organisations of every shape and size. Politics is an accepted part of everyday home and work life that you need to be aware of because it could impact on your personal career, what you are trying to achieve and your potential as a leader.

Internal politics creates a network of connections that does not exist on an organisational chart. However, those networks can be very influential, which is why knowledge of them can be important both to you as an individual and to the organisation itself. There may be internal politics between members of a team, between teams, between departments and then there is external politics which can be local or national.

With respect to internal politics, the best approach is to have a positive outlook, be authentic and professional – but don't shy away from considering other people's motives. Everyone within the work environment will have their own agenda. Some will be very upfront about what they are trying to do or what they need, whilst others may try more subtle forms of influence or persuasion. It is important that you listen to everyone and think critically about what they have said, considering not just what they are saying but what is motivating them to say or act in a certain way, so that you can balance your thinking and make up your own mind.

ACTIVITY 5.12

Can you identify an instance when internal politics affected your work? Identify what happened and consider who benefited. Why do you think politics became involved?

CHAPTER SUMMARY

Three key points to take away from Chapter 5:

- There are different sources and bases of power, an understanding of which can help you support or challenge leadership within your organisation and facilitate your emergence as a leader.

- Power and influence, and therefore leadership, can occur at any level in an organisation. Effective leaders build their power through a combination of different sources and bases, and draw on these, depending on the situation and people that they are working with.

- Politics and the influence of power on them form an inextricable part of personal and professional lives. It is important that any leader is aware of these in order to be effective in their role.

QUESTIONS

Question 5.1

What is the relationship between a source of power and a base of power? Illustrate your answer with examples from your workplace. *(Learning outcome 5.1)*

Question 5.2

Describe why words, deeds and symbols are significant in relation to power and leadership. *(Learning outcome 5.2)*

Question 5.3

Identify ways in which you can influence outcomes. *(Learning outcome 5.3)*

Question 5.4

Outline how you would recognise someone as a leader and their location within the organisation. *(Learning outcome 5.4)*

FURTHER READING

Brooks, I. (2009) *Organisational Behaviour: Individuals, Groups and Organisation*, 4th edition. Harlow: Prentice Hall.

Haslam, S.A., Reicher, S.D. & Platow, M.J. (2011) *The New Psychology of Leadership: Identity, Influence and Power.* Hove: Psychology Press.

Northcote, P.G. (2010) *Leadership: Theory and Practice*, 5th edition. California: Sage.

6

LEADERSHIP AND CHANGE MANAGEMENT

LEARNING OUTCOMES:

When you have completed this chapter you should be able to:

6.1 Discuss the meaning of change for the individual

6.2 Identify drivers for change in your organisation

6.3 Analyse the role of the leader as a catalyst for change

6.4 Give an overview of key change management models

6.5 Outline theories of motivation applied to change management

6.6 Use principled negotiation when bringing about change in practice.

INTRODUCTION

We are working in a time of considerable reform and change within our health and social care services. The reasons for this are vast and varied but centre largely on changes in society itself in terms of greater social, cultural and racial diversity; an ageing population, resulting in an increased prevalence of long-term conditions; and inequalities in health. Reforms also relate to people's higher expectations of service provision and the increased availability of technology and treatments demanding different modes of service delivery and a focus on value for money (Freshwater *et al.*, 2009). More recently, change has also been driven by the economic environment.

It is how change is managed that is crucial to its successful implementation. This chapter aims to enable you to develop an awareness of the potential impact of change on the individual and different methods of bringing about, implementing and sustaining change.

THE MEANING OF CHANGE FOR THE INDIVIDUAL

Change can bring with it wonderful opportunities for creativity, new ways of working, career development and enhanced services, to name but a few. However, it cannot be assumed that all members of your team will perceive change in this way.

> **ACTIVITY 6.1**
>
> Write a list of words that people commonly use to describe change. What percentage are positive and what percentage are negative?

A group of 43 health and social care practitioners were asked by the author to list words commonly associated with change. These are detailed in *Table 6.1*.

Table 6.1 *Words associated with change*

Frightening	Threatening	Apathetic	Resistant	Fearful
Anxious	Scared	Uncomfortable	Distrust	Unwilling
Worried	Concerned	Apprehensive	Uneasy	Fretful
Nervous	Exciting	Positive	An opportunity	Cynical

This list was compiled within one particular place of work over a 12-month period, so it may be reflective of how change was managed in that specific area. However, it is worth noting that only three of the 20 words listed are positive. In exploring with practitioners why change is often perceived so negatively, the reasons centred on change apathy and poor communication. Change apathy was linked to the scale and rate of change being perceived as too great to keep pace with and to remain enthusiastic about. In relation to communication, practitioners talked about how messages relating to change initiatives are conveyed and the negative emotions that are likely to be elicited when communication is poor and there is no room for clarification and dialogue.

Kubler-Ross's (1973) grief and loss model is frequently applied to describe people's responses to change. The model was originally developed to describe most people's emotional responses to the prospect of their own death. It describes a sequential process of denial, followed by anger, bargaining, depression and finally, with appropriate support, acceptance. Today, the model is largely accepted as being equally applicable to any significant life change.

Change may not always be perceived negatively, however. Some people readily embrace change and actively seek it out. Factors such as the way in which the change is communicated, prepared for and implemented, as well as factors that are unique to the individual such as past experiences of change, concurrent factors such as the stability of the individual's personal life, self-esteem and previous professional and academic experience will all shape the individual's perceptions. Rogers and Shoemaker (1971) classify six different categories of people who are involved in change:

- Innovators: individual team members who are excited by new ideas and are eager to implement them

- Early adopters: individuals within the team who take a few days to think about the change and then go on to adopt the change

- Early majority: several team members adopt the idea

- Later majority: a number of the team accept and take up the idea

- Laggards: individual team members who have a tendency to lag behind in accepting and adopting change

- Rejecters: individuals who usually oppose new ideas and are against change.

Gopee and Galloway (2009) suggest that understanding how people may respond to change may help in the change management process. For instance, the energy and positivity of the *innovators* can be utilised and responsibilities can be delegated to them. The *later majority* may need time to make sense of the proposed change and to pilot it. *Laggards* may need additional time and support and *rejecters* may require some additional input to identify the reasons for such opposition.

DRIVERS FOR CHANGE

In any organisation there are numerous factors that drive change. These may be at the micro level where changes may originate from the client, the unit or the department; the meso level which includes the health and/or social care organisation and the community; or the macro level which is affected by national policy. It is very important to identify where changes are coming from so that their worth or applicability can be evaluated and their purpose communicated to others.

ACTIVITY 6.2

Think of a change that you are or have been involved in; this may be in your place of work, on placement or at your university. Identify the factors that are driving that change.

An example of change that has affected the entire multi-disciplinary team over recent years is discharge planning from hospital and intermediate care. The macro drivers for this change have included guidance from the Department of Health (Department of Health, 2003b; 2004; 2010b). Meso drivers may have included key performance indicators for waiting times for patients requiring admission to hospital and intermediate care and/or community dissatisfaction. Micro drivers may include staff dissatisfaction or complaints.

One method of identifying the forces for and against a change is through force field analysis. Force field analysis is a tool that was developed by Lewin (1947) to evaluate the forces for and against a change. Each force for and against will differ in power, or force, which is represented by the length and width of the arrows (see *Figure 6.1*). For any change initiative to be successful, the forces that are driving change must be stronger than the forces resisting it.

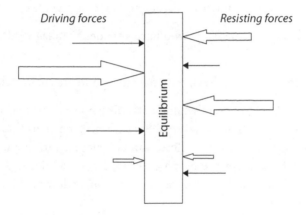

Figure 6.1 *Driving and resisting forces (adapted from Lewin, 1947)*

The resistant forces may centre on the availability of physical resources and finance, but often they will centre on the psychological reactions of the people who are involved in the change. Although the most visible symbol of change is a physical change (e.g. a move to a new building), significant changes to working practices are accompanied by social and psychological change. It is therefore essential, as a leader, to try to understand more about what underpins an individual's resistance to change. Nevis (1989) describes four sources of resistance:

- A reluctance to give up something that the individual values

- A lack of understanding of the change and its implications

- A lack of belief in the change itself, in terms of its benefits for the organisation

- A low tolerance of change.

Through being aware of all of the resisting forces it is often possible to address these and minimise them through discussing and addressing the salient points.

ACTIVITY 6.3

Now think of a change that you would like to make in practice. Use *Figure 6.1* to identify the factors that will drive the change forward as well as the resisting forces.

Another important purpose of identifying drivers for change is to ensure that the 'right' change is being made. In a busy environment, with multiple demands being made on the leader, it is easy for a change to be suggested in response to an event, with the underpinning issues that led to the event being overlooked. One way of avoiding this is the 'five whys'. This method of identifying the root cause of an issue originated within the manufacturing company Toyota, as it developed its Lean working practices to remove waste and streamline production (Bicheno, 2006). Since the 1990s Lean principles have become increasingly applied to health and social care throughout the UK in a bid to make services more efficient. Repeatedly asking the question 'why?' enables the team to establish the root cause of the issue.

The NHS Institute for Innovation and Improvement (2008) suggests that the 'five whys' are used in the following way:

- First, outline the problem by writing it down. This will help the team to clarify and focus on the problem.

- Then go on to brainstorm why the problem occurs, making a written note of the answer.

- It is likely that this answer will not fully identify the source of the problem, in which case 'why?' needs to be asked again and the answer recorded.

- This last stage may need to be repeated until the team has identified the root cause of the problem. In reality, this may take more or less than five 'whys'.

This approach is a simple method that not only helps in identifying the root cause of a problem, but also in discovering relationships between the various issues that underpin it. It also ensures that change is not directed at dealing with the symptoms, rather than addressing the problem itself (NHS Institute for Innovation and Improvement, 2008).

An example of the 'five whys' being used in a real situation is given in *Table 6.2*.

Table 6.2 *An example of the 'five whys' being used in practice*

Patients from one ward are consistently late in getting to the physiotherapy gym, causing delays for all other patients. Why?
There is a long wait for a wheelchair. Why?
Only one wheelchair on the ward works. Why?
The other wheelchairs have parts missing from them. Why?
They have not been regularly maintained. Why?
There is no maintenance schedule for wheelchairs on the ward.

THE LEADER AS A CATALYST FOR CHANGE

ACTIVITY 6.4

Identify a leader that you have seen successfully bring about, implement and sustain a change. What skills and qualities did the leader use in order to manage change effectively?

The change agent can be any person within a team or an external party charged with bringing about and implementing an agreed change, as illustrated in the scenarios below.

SCENARIO 6.1

An inquiry following revelations of unsafe restraint practices in an NHS Trust recommended that an external body be brought in to review and change practice. The external body was given 12 weeks by the Trust to fulfil this brief. Contrary to the expectations of staff, initially the external agents concentrated their energies on eliciting staff opinions of what the main issues were. They also spent time discussing how staff felt about their continuing professional development needs. Slowly a relationship of trust developed and the agents' track record in the field and professionalism earned them the respect of the staff. They helped staff to become aware of best practice in the field and helped them to take ownership by enabling the staff to plan how they would implement the guidance. An action plan was drawn up by the staff and implemented by the end of the twelfth week.

SCENARIO 6.2

Heidi works at a playgroup, which meets every morning in a community hall to allow pre-school children to play and learn together. Heidi became a member of staff three years ago, having worked at several full-time nurseries prior to this. Heidi's initial impressions of the playgroup were that the practices were rather rigid and could be more child-focused. This view was supported by a recent Ofsted report. However, Heidi was mindful that most of the staff had worked there for many years. She kept her views to herself and focused on demonstrating her competence through her work with the children. After nine months she gently introduced new ideas for play, always discussing her rationale and ensuring that the staff were happy with her ideas. She then enrolled at the local university to start a course in early years studies. Heidi slowly gained the trust and respect of her colleagues and several followed her example in undertaking academic study. Heidi's job title and status did not change; at no point was she the formal leader or manager. However, in time, staff allowed her to introduce further change to reflect modern-day thinking in the area. The playgroup now enjoys a good reputation and is considered by both Ofsted and parents to offer excellent educational opportunities for pre-school children.

ACTIVITY 6.5

Review the list of qualities and skills that you identified in *Activity 6.4*. Now that you have read the above examples, develop your list further.

Your responses to *Activity 6.4* probably mirrored many of the skills and qualities discussed in *Chapter 3*, such as effective communication, emotional intelligence and a knowledge of the field. However, the scenarios highlight other, equally important issues to be considered when acting as an agent of change.

Both of the scenarios above placed a great deal of emphasis on trust. A good relationship and mutual trust between the agent of change and those that he or she works with is more likely to elicit a positive response to new ways of thinking and working (NHS Institute for Innovation and Improvement, 2005b). Scholtes (1998) argues that trust is elicited from a combination of competency and caring, as illustrated in *Figure 6.2*. Competency on its own will bring about respect but not trust. Equally, if the individual feels cared for by the change agent but does not consider the leader to be competent or capable, it is likely that the individual will have affection for that person but may not trust them.

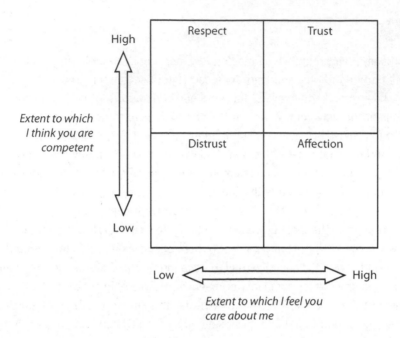

Figure 6.2 *Competency, caring and trust (adapted from Scholtes, 1998)*

Transformational leadership is also a feature of the above two examples. As discussed in *Chapter 2*, transformational leadership is widely held to be suited to environments where change is constant (Welford, 2002; Thyer, 2003; NHS Confederation, 1999). This is because of its emphasis on individualised consideration, people's emotions, intrinsic motivation, follower development, shared values and long-term goals, all of which are pivotal to bringing about and sustaining change. In *Scenario 6.2*, Heidi also acted as a role model in order to influence others and bring about change. Role-modelling is an aspect of transformational leadership that can yield personal power on the part of the leader.

Northouse (2010) outlines the importance of the transformational leader in bringing about change but also emphasises the interdependency of the follower and leader in the transformational process. Bass (1985) asserts that transformational leadership alone is inadequate if it is not combined with transactional methods of leadership. Both *Scenarios 6.1* and *6.2* outlined a link to established standards and all parties involved would have been aware that to adhere to safety standards and Ofsted guidance was in their best interests. It could therefore be argued that although at face value the dominant leadership style was transformational, transactional leadership was a less obvious feature.

CHANGE MANAGEMENT MODELS

Beckhard and Harris's change equation

You have already started to formalise your own ideas around the 'best way' to bring about change. Over the last 60 years numerous theorists have developed systematic approaches to change, also known as change management models. One of the simplest approaches to change management that has been widely embraced by industry, governments and health and social care is Beckhard and Harris's change model, also known as the change equation (Beckhard & Harris, 1987). The model places staff involvement in the change process at its heart. The authors assert that in order to overcome resistance to change (R), three components of change need to be addressed: dissatisfaction (D) with the present situation, a vision (V) of what is possible and the first steps (F) that can be taken towards the vision. This is presented as:

$$D \times V \times F > R$$

In line with fundamental mathematical principles, if one of the three components is not addressed and therefore yields zero, the resistance to change will dominate. The model is of use, both when planning the change to ensure that the three elements are addressed and also during the change, as a problem solving tool to establish why resistance to the change may be occurring.

ACTIVITY 6.6

Refer back to the change that you identified in *Activity 6.3*. How would you apply the change equation to your particular change?

Dissatisfaction with the present situation can help the team recognise the need for change. To create dissatisfaction, it may be that the patient's or client's perspective needs to be considered. For example, when one Trust was moving over to a different catering model for in-patients, staff were asked to experience meal times as the patients did. This helped staff realise that meals were cold and barely palatable by the time they reached the patient, and so a different system was required. Alternatively, the team's perspective may be relevant. For example, in promoting new methods of manual handling, a review of back injuries and associated absenteeism within the team may promote a sense of dissatisfaction with the status quo. Other perspectives may include those of employers, governing bodies, statutory services and relatives.

In articulating a vision of the future it needs to be described in a way that is clear for everyone in the team to envision. The individual's ability to picture the change may be influenced by their individual learning style and thus all learning styles need to be appealed to when discussing the vision for change with the team. Honey and Mumford (1986) outline four main learning styles:

Activists are generally open-minded and happy to try anything new, with a tendency to act first and think later. They are inclined to thrive on the challenge of new experiences but become bored with the implementation and longer-term consolidation.

Reflectors like time to think, research and observe from various perspectives before reaching a conclusion. They generally adopt a low profile and when they act it is underpinned by reference to the past as well as the present and observations of others.

Theorists integrate observations into coherent theories. They are analytical and are inclined to be perfectionists who work to ensure that everything fits into a rational scheme. They are consistently logical and feel uneasy with subjective judgements and lateral thinking.

Pragmatists are keen to test new ideas and techniques to see if they work in practice. They are practical in their focus and actively seek out new ideas. They like to get on with things quickly when ideas attract them and can be impatient with open-ended debates.

The first steps of the project (F) need to be outlined to the team so that they can prepare themselves for the change (e.g. upskilling) and understand their contribution to the change.

Lewin's three-stage process of change

Lewin's three-stage process of change (Lewin, 1951) is a particularly well-known model of change. The model advocates a planned approach to change using three stages: 'unfreezing', 'movement' and 'refreezing':

- 'Unfreezing' is concerned with enabling the team to recognise the need for change and challenging and reducing the forces which support established ways of working.

- 'Movement' is the phase where new attitudes and/or behaviours are developed and the organisation moves through the various stages of implementation of the change.

- 'Refreezing' is characterised by ensuring that the change is sustained. The change is reinforced through supportive mechanisms, such as coaching, appropriate policies and organisational norms.

ACTIVITY 6.7

A recent audit of care delivery in a residential home revealed that bathroom doors were consistently left open by staff when clients were being washed and bathed. How could Lewin's model of change be applied to enhance the dignity of clients in the home?

Methods of 'unfreezing' may include staff working together to consider a SWOT analysis (p. 117) and a force field analysis (p. 80). In addressing restraining forces in the force field analysis, it may be that staff need to be facilitated in perceiving the issue from the residents' perspective. Relevant key performance indicators may also be considered as a driving force. A mixture of transformational and transactional leadership will be required (Bass, 1985) due to the need to bring about new ways of working, coupled with key performance indicators concerning dignity. In implementing the change issues such as planning, the learning culture of the organisation, education, resources, methods of overcoming resistance, communication and ongoing evaluation will all be pivotal. 'Refreezing' is often overlooked in practice. In this example, methods of ensuring that the changed behaviour is sustained could be through providing ongoing education, monitoring mechanisms, staff retaining ownership of the change and ongoing leadership support.

Kotter's eight-step change model

Kotter's eight-step change model (Kotter, 1996) offers further insight into understanding and managing change. Each stage highlights a key principle that focuses on people's responses and approaches to change. The eight steps are:

- Create urgency

- Build a team to bring about the change

- Construct the vision

- Communicate the vision for buy-in

- Empower individuals to execute the change

- Use short-term goals and reward the achievement of these

- Maintain persistence

- Sustain the change.

Cummings and Worley's six guidelines for cultural change

Cummings and Worley (2005) propose six guidelines specifically for cultural change that have parallels with Kotter's eight-step change model. The six stages are:

- Devise and articulate a clear strategic vision

- Display a willingness to change on the part of senior management

- Model the cultural change at the highest level within the organisation

- Alter the organisation to support organisational change

- Select and socialise newcomers and bypass those who do not fit in

- Develop an understanding of the ethical and legal issues that may arise as a result of the cultural change.

ACTIVITY 6.8

Compare Cummings and Worley's (2005) guidelines for cultural change with Kotter's eight-step change model (Kotter, 1996). What are the strengths and weaknesses of each model?

Prochaska and DiClemente's trans-theoretical model

The trans-theoretical (stages of change) model (Prochaska & DiClemente, 2005) is largely used as an approach to behavioural change in the context of lifestyle changes. However, more recently the model has been adopted by some organisations to bring about and implement change in a variety of settings. The model is based on observations that people engage in a series of actions or stages when making behavioural changes. These are influenced by cognitive, affective, evaluative and behaviourally orientated processes. The stages of change are:

- **Pre-contemplation** – the person does not intend to make any changes. They may not be motivated or they may be resistant to change.

- **Contemplation** – the individual contemplates and expresses a desire for change.

- **Preparation** – the person expresses a clear intention to change.

- **Action** – the individual starts to change their behaviour.

- **Maintenance** – the individual achieves and is maintaining their change.

At each stage, interventions are put in place to help the individual move from one stage to the next.

ACTIVITY 6.9

How could the trans-theoretical model (Prochaska & DiClemente, 2005) be applied to change in your practice setting?

MOTIVATIONAL THEORY

All of the change models outlined are concerned with movement from the current state to the desired state. To facilitate this process, team motivation is vital. There are several theories of motivation, all of which focus on the relationship between attitudes, needs and behaviours (Huber, 2010).

ACTIVITY 6.10

What motivates people? How could this knowledge be applied to bringing about change in your organisation?

One of the best known theories of motivation is that of Abraham Maslow (Maslow, 1954). The principle of Maslow's theory of motivation is that as humans we have needs that dominate our attention until they are satisfied. There is a hierarchy of needs that begins with our fundamental biological and physiological needs, such as the need for food and fluids. Our needs are ordered in a hierarchical framework, moving up to safety needs, followed by esteem needs, then belongingness and love, and culminating in 'self-actualisation'. It is only when a lower level need is satisfied that an employee will be motivated by the opportunity of having the next need in the hierarchy satisfied. This theory is particularly salient at the moment with many health and social care employees being concerned about their 'safety needs' in relation to the realignment of services and concerns they have about their job security. Maslow's theory suggests that if job security is threatened, then motivating individuals towards affiliation with others, which is so important in cultural change (Cummings and Worley, 2005), may be problematic.

McClelland (1987) identifies three types of motivational need:

- achievement motivation
- authority/power motivation
- affiliation motivation.

Each of these can be appealed to throughout the change cycle, with different aspects of the process being highlighted to different individuals, depending upon their motivational needs. For example, somebody who values affiliation may be motivated to engage in a particular change project in order to cultivate relationships, in which case this aspect of the project can be emphasised during the planning stage of the change process.

Herzberg's (1968) motivational theory asserts that satisfaction and dissatisfaction at work nearly always arise from different factors. He demonstrated that certain factors truly motivate people ('motivators'), whereas others ('hygiene factors') only temporarily drive them. People are unhappy if their hygiene needs are not met but once they are satisfied, the sense of satisfaction is only temporary. His work therefore suggests that people will not be 'motivated' by the satisfaction of 'hygiene' needs.

'Motivators' include a sense of achievement, recognition, the work itself, responsibility, advancement and personal growth. 'Hygiene factors' or 'maintenance factors' centre on status, security, company policy and administration, supervision, personal life, salary, work conditions and relationships with subordinates, peers and supervisor. All of the 'motivators' can be readily addressed throughout the change process, as long as the leadership style is sufficiently sensitive to allow for this. 'Hygiene factors' may be more difficult to control and need to be taken into account when expecting people to engage in change.

NEGOTIATING SKILLS

Most changes will require some degree of negotiation. Successful negotiation leads to an outcome which both parties are fully committed to and feel they benefit from. Principled negotiation (Fisher & Ury, 1981) is widely regarded as an ethical and productive approach to negotiation.

The process begins with those engaged in the negotiation defining the issue or problem together. The first principle is 'Separate the people from the problem'. The aim is to be resolute with the problem but respectful to the individuals involved in the discussions. For example, if the problem is that an adequate supply of equipment is not consistently available in a department, the normal line that the discussion may take is to blame the staff who have placed the order. The discussions may even become personal. However, in separating out the people from the problem, the processes will be focused on rather than the individual. That is not to say that staff are not accountable for their actions, but they are treated with respect and the issue is explored from all angles. The second principle is 'Focus on interests, not positions'. Taking up a particular position, for example 'I will only accept...', 'I will not...' will often lead to an impasse. However, even when opposed positions are adopted there are often still shared and compatible interests which can be explored, for example the desire to deliver a high quality service. To identify interests, questions such as 'why?' and 'why not?' can be effective. The third principle, 'Invent options for mutual gain', is something that can be explored prior to meeting; however, this process can also be beneficial if carried out within the negotiations. In looking for 'mutual gain' it can be beneficial to identify shared interests. The fourth principle, 'Insist on objective criteria', requires preparation in that the 'objective criteria' may be concerned with professional standards, accepted practice, the evidence base, efficiency, costs, law and ethical standards, which may need to be explored in some detail.

CONFLICT MANAGEMENT

Whilst conflict can be an energising force, if handled badly it can be destructive. Conflict management strategies involve preventing the conflict from escalating, containing the conflict and addressing the conflict (NHS Institute for Innovation and Improvement, 2005b). Gerzon (2006) proposes that the leader can address conflict effectively and transform differences into opportunities through eight tools:

- *Integral vision*: the leader addresses all sides of the conflict.

- *Systems thinking*: the leader identifies the various elements of the issue and how they work together.

- *Presence*: the leader visibly applies him/herself mentally and emotionally to the conflict situation.

- *Inquiry*: the leader asks questions of all parties to elicit information to provide an understanding of how to transform the situation.

- *Conscious conversation*: the leader is mindful of their communication and listening skills.

- *Dialogue*: communication is used to bridge and innovate.

- *Bridging*: partnerships are created that transcend the barriers that divide the parties.

- *Innovation*: methods of addressing conflicts that create new ways of dealing with conflicts are fostered.

However, each of us will vary in our approach to managing conflict. The Thomas–Kilmann conflict mode instrument (Kilmann, 2010) outlines five different modes for responding to conflict situations:

- Competing

- Accommodating

- Avoiding

- Collaborating

- Compromising.

Each of us is capable of using all five conflict-handling modes. Our response to conflict will depend upon our personal predispositions and the requirements of the conflict situation. People rarely have a single style of dealing with conflict, but we may have a tendency to rely on certain modes more than on others. An awareness of our natural tendencies can be helpful in enhancing our responses to conflict which may occur as part of the process of change.

> **CHAPTER SUMMARY**
>
> **Three key points to take away from Chapter 6:**
>
> ↪ Change management requires real sensitivity, taking into account individuals' past experiences of change, the meaning that they attach to the change and their level of motivation. An awareness of these factors will allow for appropriate strategies to be put in place to support individuals to engage in the change process.
>
> ↪ Any change will have driving forces that support its implementation. Through being aware of these one is able to evaluate whether the proposals are 'right' for the organisation and potential resisting forces can be identified and addressed.
>
> ↪ Transformational leadership is pivotal in bringing about and sustaining change; however, this may need to be coupled with transactional leadership depending upon the context.

QUESTIONS

Question 6.1

Outline the potential meanings of change for the individual. *(Learning outcome 6.1)*

Question 6.2

What are the drivers for change in your organisation? *(Learning outcome 6.2)*

Question 6.3

What is the leader's role in bringing about change? *(Learning outcome 6.3)*

Question 6.4

Name and describe the change management models that you have explored in this chapter. *(Learning outcome 6.4)*

Question 6.5

Outline three theories of motivation that can be applied to change management. *(Learning outcome 6.5)*

Question 6.6

What is principled negotiation and how is it carried out? *(Learning outcome 6.6)*

FURTHER READING

Fisher, R. & Ury, W. (1981) *Getting to Yes. Negotiating Agreement Without Giving In.* London: Hutchinson Business.

Gerzon, M. (2006) *Leading Through Conflict. How Successful Leaders Transform Differences into Opportunities.* Boston: Harvard Business School Press.

7

LEADERSHIP IN HEALTH AND SOCIAL CARE

LEARNING OUTCOMES:

When you have completed this chapter you should be able to:

7.1 Describe the macro structure and function of the NHS and care services

7.2 Summarise key government changes and policies

7.3 Understand the changing role of service users and carers and the impact of this on services

7.4 Describe how the locus of leadership is changing in the NHS and care services.

INTRODUCTION

So far you have been considering leadership theory and the different aspects of organisational life which impact on how an individual undertakes a leadership role. This chapter moves on to introduce you to the context in which you are working within the health and social care sector.

Recent years have seen many changes in both the health and care services, and in the people and professions that staff them. Some of these changes have been driven by local or regional needs, or by developments within the professions themselves. However, the majority of changes have related to developments in government policy. Another key factor in the current structures within the health and care environment relates directly to the transfer of powers, including those relating to health and social care, to the Northern

Ireland Assembly, Scottish Parliament and Welsh Assembly, following devolution from the Westminster Parliament in 1998/9. There has also been a significant change in the power relationship between patients/clients/service users and the health or social care staff who work with them. This again links to changes in policy but also to advances in technology. As was identified in *Chapter 1*, there has also been a change in the locus of leadership within both the NHS and care services, with far more distributed leadership coming to the fore.

THE NHS AND CARE SERVICES – HOW WE GOT TO WHERE WE ARE

ACTIVITY 7.1

Consider the organisation you are currently working in. When and why was it established?

Health and care organisations have changed significantly over the years. There are many factors that have influenced these changes, amongst which are social, economic, political and technological developments. It is not essential that you know fully about these changes; however, an understanding will help you appreciate how we got to where we are today. Some of the changes in the way health and care services have been delivered, or the reports/policies/bills which have affected them, are outlined below. These brief histories are by no means exhaustive; they simply touch on some of the factors which may help you better understand the context of the current environment in which you are working and emerging as a leader.

A BRIEF HISTORY OF THE NHS

The NHS was established in 1948 in the aftermath of the Second World War when health care was a luxury that not everyone could afford. It involved the nationalisation of all hospitals, voluntary or state, and the setting up of a regional framework. It was based on the principles that everyone was eligible for care, provision of care was entirely free at the point of use (although prescription and dental charges were later brought in) and funded through taxation. It was run by the Ministry of Health and had three elements: hospital services, community health services and local authority services. In 1962 the 10-year Hospital Plan was published, which proposed the development of district general hospitals all over the country. Between 1968 and 1974 there was much debate over how the NHS should be organised. Key issues included local government reorganisation (see Seebohm in Social Care history, below) and the desire to improve the coordination of health and social services.

In 1974 the NHS was reorganised into 14 Regional Health Authorities and a new tier of Area Health Authorities (AHA) was established. Boundaries were largely coterminous between the AHAs and local authorities to enable coordination across the two; however, the system was very complex and very managerially driven. Towards the early 1980s it became evident that the NHS funding available was not sufficient to deliver everything that technology and medical advances could offer. Restructuring took place again in 1982 and AHAs were abolished. General management was introduced in 1984 and there began to be an increasing emphasis on management and leadership.

In 1989 there was a further, fundamental review of the whole NHS which led to the publication of a White Paper, *Working for Patients*, which passed into law as the NHS and Community Care Act (1990). This established an 'internal' market and enabled 'purchasers' (health authorities and some family doctors) to buy health from 'providers' (acute hospitals, organisations providing care for the mentally ill, the elderly and ambulance services). To gain 'provider' status, health organisations became NHS trusts; independent organisations which competed against one another for business. The wider issues of the country's health were reviewed in the *Health of the Nation* (Department of Health, 1992) which identified health promotion as an area for growth. By 1995 all health care was provided by trusts and some GPs were given budgets with which to buy health care; however, there were tensions in the system due to inequalities for patients of fund-holding versus non-fund-holding GPs, and in 1997 a new White Paper was issued, *The New NHS: Modern, Dependable* (Department of Health, 1997), and again restructuring was proposed.

In 1998/9 power in relation to health and social care was transferred from the Westminster Parliament to the Northern Ireland Assembly, Scottish Parliament and Welsh Assembly. This led to changes in the landscape of health services as political devolution enabled the different countries to develop their own responses to the health challenges that they faced. The way in which they planned, organised and managed their health services started to diverge; however, the basic principles on which the NHS was founded were retained (Jervis & Plowden, 2003). The divergence was also affected by the funding system, as the devolved nations receive funding from the UK Treasury in a block grant determined by the Barnett formula. A simple example of this divergence is seen in the Welsh Assembly's decision that prescriptions should be free in Wales from 2007. Northern Ireland followed suit in 2010 and Scotland in 2011.

In England, the NHS Plan (Department of Health, 2000b) saw further restructuring in England, leading to the formation of 10 Strategic Health Authorities and around 200 Primary Care Trusts contracted with both public and private providers for a wide range of services, as well as GPs. At this time NICE, the National Institute for Clinical Excellence (as it was then termed) was established, which assessed the cost-effectiveness of new drugs and treatments. Payment by results was introduced and cost-effectiveness and affordability came to the fore. Independent treatment centres and NHS walk-in centres were introduced, as was competition between providers of care. The Wanless Report (Department of Health,

2002) looked at how the NHS was performing against public expectations and took an evidence-based view of the resources that would be needed by the NHS over the following 20 years. A further review, the *Next Stage Review* (Department of Health, 2007), was undertaken by Lord Darzi, and quality was made central to NHS development in England. Clinical advances continued to accelerate, although the global financial crisis meant substantial change for the NHS again and a further restructuring of the NHS in England was proposed in the White Paper *Equity and Excellence: Liberating the NHS* (Department of Health, 2010a).

In Scotland, *Our National Health: A Plan for Action, a Plan for Change* (Scottish Executive, 2000) and the Community Care and Health (Scotland) Act (Scottish Executive, 2002) signalled a significant shift in the approach to health services. The internal market was abolished, NHS Health Boards were created and the number of NHS Trusts halved, with the new structure being based on collaboration rather than competition. The publication of *Improving Health in Scotland: The Challenge* (Scottish Executive, 2003) proposed a strategic framework to support the health improvement of people in Scotland, recognising the country's specific health issues. This was followed in 2005 by the final Kerr report *Building a Health Service Fit for the Future* (Scottish Executive, 2005). *Better Health, Better Care* (Scottish Executive, 2007) then set the direction of travel for healthcare services and acted as the foundation for *The NHS Scotland Quality Strategy* (Scottish Executive, 2010).

A plan for the NHS in Wales, *Improving Health in Wales: A Plan for the NHS with its Partners* (NHS Wales, 2001), proposed new structures and organisational change building on the earlier *Better Health, Better Wales* (NHS Wales, 1998a) and *Putting Patients First* (NHS Wales, 1998b). Amongst other changes, it led to the dissolution of the five Health Authorities and the creation of a Health and Social Care Department, with three regional offices and 21 Local Health Boards. In 2005 the Welsh Assembly published *Designed for Life* (Welsh Assembly Government, 2005) which set out a strategic framework for working towards the establishment of world class health and social care services over the next 10 years. In 2009 a reorganisation of NHS Wales came into effect which created single local health organisations responsible for delivering all services in a geographical area rather than the previous Trust and Local Health Board system. It also ended the internal NHS market. *Together for Health* (NHS Wales, 2011) then set out a five-year vision for the NHS in Wales to achieve better health for everyone. It indicated the intention to establish a number of centres of excellence whilst recognising the importance of community-based services.

Changes in the NHS in Northern Ireland moved at a different pace to those in Scotland and Wales due to the stopping and starting of the devolution process. In addition, Northern Ireland is unique in that it shares a border with an EU member rather than one of the UK nations. This has meant a different focus on health and care than in other countries. The *Investing for Health Strategy* (Department of Health, Social Services and Public Safety, 2002) set out to improve the health and wellbeing of the people of Northern Ireland and reduce health inequalities through an increased focus on prevention. Recommendations from the *Review of Public Administration* (RPA, 2003) and the *Independent Review of Health and Social Services Care in Northern Ireland* (Appleby, 2005) were built upon and led to the restructuring of services outlined in the Health and Social Care (Reform) Act (Department of Health, Social Services and Public Safety, 2009), which included the creation of a single Health and Social Care Board. It should be noted that there has always been greater integration of health and social care in Northern Ireland than in the other parts of the UK. *Transforming Your Care* (Department of Health, Social Services and Public Safety, 2011) proposed a new model of integrated care with Integrated Care Partnerships and an increased focus on the individual.

A BRIEF HISTORY OF SOCIAL CARE SERVICES

Social welfare systems in one form or another have existed for several centuries; however, contemporary social care services are considered to have begun after the Second World War with a raft of 'Welfare State' initiatives and services such as residential care and a range of children's services being provided under legislation such as the National Assistance Act (HMSO, 1948). These 'traditional' professional-led services continued, mainly separately, as specialist Departments until the Seebohm Report (1968) and the Health Services and Public Health Act (HMSO, 1968) created social services departments which were generic and served 'whole families / communities'. This system, with social workers having a mix of elderly, young and mental health cases continued until the Children Act (HMSO, 1989) and the National Health Service and Community Care Act (HMSO, 1990), after which social services departments had to become less generic as their work became more specialised, scrutinised and legally challenged. The introduction of 'Best Value' in the late 1980s posed a more extensive, challenging and comprehensive performance regime than anything that had been attempted before.

Differences emerged between the four nations of the UK following devolution, in relation to structures, policies and regulation (Birrell, 2007). For example, in Scotland the reorganisation of local government led to some social work departments being merged with housing, while some children's services merged with education. The publication of *For Scotland's Children* (Scottish Executive, 2001a) led to increased integration between health education and social services. The Scottish Social Services Council was established under the Regulation of Care (Scotland) Act (Scottish Executive, 2001b) with the remit to improve the quality and standards of social services and so increase public protection. *Changing Lives: Report of the 21st Century Social Work Review* (Scottish Executive, 2006) set a new direction for social work services based on core values of inclusiveness and meeting the whole needs of individuals and families. It focused on building capacity to deliver personalised services, the capacity of the workforce itself and on making these changes sustainable. However, one of the biggest policy changes following devolution was the provision of free personal care for older people, whether they were in the community or in a residential home or a nursing home, in the Community Care and Health (Scotland) Act (Scottish Executive, 2002).

In Northern Ireland, the *Review of Public Administration* (RPA, 2003) and the *Independent Review of Health and Social Services Care in Northern Ireland* (Appleby, 2005) led to the increasing integration of social services with health services. Five new integrated Health and Social Care Trusts were established in 2007 and then later a regional Health and Social Care Board was set up to replace the four Health and Social Services Boards. The restructuring of services, outlined in the Health and Social Care (Reform) Act (Department of Health, Social Services and Public Safety, 2009), also included a Patient and Client Council. This was set up to replace the Health and Social Services Councils to ensure service users and carers had a strong voice. *Transforming Your Care* (Department of Health, Social Services and Public Safety, 2011) proposed significant changes to the way services were to be delivered, with a new, improved model of delivery based around Integrated Care Partnerships.

In Wales, modernisation of services was based on improving collaboration rather than competition, an approach which was outlined in *Making Connections: delivering better services for Wales* (Welsh Assembly Government, 2004) and built on in *Designed for Life* (Welsh Assembly Government, 2005) and the *Beyond Boundaries* review (Beecham, 2006). In particular, the Welsh Assembly made high quality services for older people a priority to prolong wellbeing and facilitate independent living. In 2006 Wales introduced the Social Services Improvement Agency to support and improve Local Authority services for both adults and children. In 2007 *Fulfilled Lives, Supportive Communities* (Welsh Assembly Government, 2007) was published, which outlined the strategy for modernising social services in Wales over the next 10 years. In the same year, the Social Services Inspectorate for Wales and the Care Standards Inspectorate for Wales were amalgamated to make a combined Care and Social Services Inspectorate to ensure a more integrated approach to social services and care. In 2009 they introduced an overarching framework for local authority social services inspection, review and evaluation, which was intended to be citizen focused and to encourage improvement and innovation as well as integration.

In England, 'modernised' social care services can be seen to have begun more specifically with the publication of the White Paper *Modernising Social Services: Promoting Independence, Improving Protection, Raising Standards* (Department of Health, 1998), which set out a vision for personal social services. The White Paper *Modern Local Government: In Touch with the People* (Department of the Environment, Transport and the Regions, 1998) stipulated that constant improvement in both quality and cost would be expected from local government, with 'Best Value' becoming a statutory duty from 1st April 2000. In the process, the three 'e's were emphasised: '[Best Value] is a statutory duty to deliver services taking into account quality and cost by the most effective, economic and efficient means possible' (HMSO, 1999, Annex A). Over a five-year period, all local authority services were subjected to Best Value reviews and Best Value performance plans were drawn up. Not only was social work included in this far-reaching evaluative activity, but it was also linked specifically to Best Value through requirements to deliver services to clear standards, paying attention to quality and cost and demonstrating a commitment to continuous improvement in the efficiency and effectiveness of its performance (Department of Health, 1998). Thus, the 'modernisation' of social work was rooted in the Best Value regime and demonstrated through the implementation of national performance standards and targets. Performance elements were set out in the *Quality Strategy for Social Care 2000* (Department of Health, 2000a) and included national service frameworks, national standards, service models, and local performance measures against which progress within an agreed timescale would be monitored.

POLICIES AND STRATEGIES

The devolution of many government activities, including the transfer of power in relation to health and social care in 1998/9 from the Westminster Parliament to the Northern Ireland Assembly, Scottish Parliament and Welsh Assembly led to the creation of a number of country-specific policies. The backbone for the majority of health and social care provision, however, remains the UK-wide policies that were in existence up until the point of devolution. In addition, changes in England, the largest of the four countries within the UK, still influence provision in the other countries.

Each government produces a number of papers, strategies and frameworks which are modified over the years due to changing political and contextual circumstances. When looking at resources in this area, it is very important to recognise that policy introduced initially to an assembly or parliament in one year may take several months or potentially years to be fully implemented. Each country has a defined process which has to be followed in order to ensure democracy is upheld. Examples pertaining to each of the four countries in the UK can be found through the following websites:

*   www.dh.gov.uk

*   www.niassembly.gov.uk

*   www.scotland.gov.uk

*   www.wales.nhs.gov.uk

WHY IS KNOWLEDGE OF GOVERNMENT POLICY IMPORTANT?

The power of knowledge and the importance of influence were both raised in *Chapter 5* as being key to effective leadership. With the current pace and complexity of change occurring in the health and social care arena, it is more important than ever to have an understanding of the different organisations involved in the commissioning, delivering and monitoring of health and care services to ensure that you hold meaningful conversations with the right people. In an increasingly competitive and busy world, being able to prioritise your time and energy effectively will be crucial in gaining respect as a leader as well as achieving successful outcomes for your organisation.

A good example of how a change in policy can lead to significant changes arose from the publication of the White Paper *Equity and Excellence: Liberating the NHS* (Department of Health, 2010a), which affected both health and social care in England. The government identified clearly that it maintained a commitment to an NHS that was available to all, free at the point of use and based on need and not the ability to pay – fundamental founding principles. However, although the government committed itself to an increase in health spending in real terms, the White Paper acknowledged the financial environment current in 2010 and the need for NHS organisations to make unprecedented efficiency gains in order to meet the costs of demographic and technological changes.

The White Paper outlined fundamental reforms of the structure and delivery of NHS services in England. The reforms were based on the government's stated core beliefs of freedom, fairness and responsibility. They identified that the intention of the White Paper was to make the NHS more accountable to patients, put patients at the heart of the NHS and focus on outcomes and empowering health professionals. They confirmed that their vision for the NHS was one which:

- centred on service users and carers
- could demonstrate quality and outcomes amongst the best in the world
- eliminated discrimination and inequalities in care
- put clinicians in the driving seat and enabled hospitals and providers to innovate and adopt best practice
- was more transparent in respect of quality and results
- was less fragmented with better cross-boundary working, particularly between local authorities, hospitals and practices
- was more efficient and dynamic, with much less national, regional and local bureaucracy.

ACTIVITY 7.2

Reflecting on the points above, identify why strong leadership is going to be important in the delivery of these outcomes.

Making significant changes to the way services are delivered and increasing working across health and care boundaries, in addition to enhancing the role of frontline practitioners in making things happen are all things which can only be achieved through excellent leadership and joined-up thinking. Leaders are needed with the vision to see how they can best work with colleagues to ensure their piece of the health and care 'jigsaw' has the best possible fit with other pieces of the jigsaw. Together the different leaders need to ensure that the jigsaw is made complete in a way that makes sense for service users and carers. With the level of change proposed, the need for strong leadership is particularly important; to deliver cohesive and transformational change is much more of a challenge than leading in a time of stability. This is also a policy where teamwork both within and across organisations is vital, and the potential for leaders at all levels of organisations to emerge is significant.

In addition, the increase in role for service users in making decisions about their care, their choice of healthcare provider and the use of personal budgets means an increased need for leadership through all levels of organisations, right down to the point of care, i.e. distributed leadership.

ACTIVITY 7.3

Identify a recent government policy relating to your area of work and outline what it has meant for your organisation.

THE STRUCTURE OF THE NHS AND SOCIAL CARE SERVICES ACROSS THE UK

This section is designed to give you a brief introduction to some of the key organisations and groups which could impact on your working life, your role as a leader and your career. Although many have their own websites, this is not always the case, so when searching for information a good starting point is always the main government website for each country, given earlier in this chapter.

England

The **Department of Health** is responsible for high level policy development. It is a complex organisation comprising a number of directorates supported by various boards and committees. It is led by the Secretary of State for Health. (www.dh.gov.uk)

Public Health England (PHE) works closely with local authorities and other partners to raise awareness of local public health issues and ensure that improved public health outcomes are delivered. It incorporates functions from the Health Protection Agency, the National Treatment Agency, the Public Health Observatories and cancer registries.

NHS Trusts are responsible for the provision and delivery of NHS services. Foundation trusts are independent legal entities with public benefit corporation status and unique governance arrangements. They are accountable to the local population that they serve. They are overseen by Monitor (see below).

The NHS Commissioning Board supports the clinical commissioning groups and is responsible for allocating and accounting for NHS resources. It also directly commissions services for certain specialist services. It is responsible for ensuring improvements in quality and extending public and patient involvement and choice. (www.healthandcare.dh.gov.uk)

Monitor is the independent regulator of Foundation Trusts. It is also the body which assesses when NHS Trusts are ready for Foundation Trust status. One of its duties is to facilitate integrated care. (www.monitor-nhsft.gov.uk)

The **Cooperation and Competition Panel (CCP)** reports to Monitor and is responsible for the assessment of 'any qualified provider' for elective NHS services. (www.ccpanel.org.uk)

Clinical commissioning groups (previously referred to as **GP consortia**) are responsible for local commissioning, supported and overseen by the NHS Commissioning Board. They work in collaboration with local authorities. They are primarily made up of GP practices; however, patients, carers, the public and a wide range of doctors, nurses and other health and care professionals are also involved in the commissioning process. They have a duty to promote integrated health and social care.

Clinical Senates provide a forum for cross-specialty clinical expertise, collaboration and advice where doctors, nurses and other professionals come together to give advice to commissioners.

Clinical Networks are linked groups of health professionals and organisations from primary, secondary and tertiary care who work together to ensure equitable provision of high-quality and clinically-effective service. They are expected to challenge existing models of care and workforce arrangements, and to improve cross-boundary working. (www. healthcareworkforce.nhs.uk)

Local Authorities are responsible for the provision of social care services. Reforms to the NHS mean that councils will be taking more responsibility for health in the community. Local authorities are able to commission local HealthWatch or HealthWatch England to provide advocacy and support. (www.nhs.uk/aboutNHSChoices)

Health and Wellbeing Boards focus on local health inequalities, addressing the broader determinants of health and wellbeing as well as improving evidence-based prevention and health and social care services for individuals.

The **Care Quality Commission (CQC)** is the regulator for care provided by the NHS, local authorities, private companies and voluntary organisations. Their aim is to make sure better care is provided for everyone, whether in hospitals, care homes or their own homes. They undertake regular inspection visits and publish reports of the findings. (www.cqc.org.uk)

HealthWatch England comes under the CQC as the independent consumer champion. They provide leadership, advice and support to local HealthWatch, as well as advocacy services. They provide advice to the NHS Commissioning Board, Monitor and the Secretary of State.

Local HealthWatch organisations ensure that the views and feedback from patients and carers are taken account of in local commissioning across health and social care. (www. advocacyresource.org.uk/HealthWatch)

The **National Institute for Health and Clinical Excellence (NICE)** makes recommendations to the NHS on new and existing medicines, treatments and procedures, and on treating and caring for people with specific diseases and conditions. It also makes recommendations to the NHS, local authorities and other organisations in the public, private, voluntary and community sectors on health improvement. (www.nice.org.uk)

Health Education England (HEE) is responsible for leading and overseeing the planning and development of the health and public health workforce, as well as for the allocation of education and training resources. Health and care providers and professionals work with HEE through Local Education and Training Boards (LETBs) to ensure and improve the quality of education and training outcomes.

ACTIVITY 7.4a

If you work in England, which of the above organisations most recently interacted with your organisation, and why?

Northern Ireland

Devolution was restored to the Northern Ireland Assembly in May 2007, which included the transfer of powers relating to health and social care services from the Westminster Parliament (www.niassembly.gov.uk). The Northern Ireland Assembly has an Executive and eleven departments, of which one is the **Department of Health, Social Services and Public Safety** (www.dhsspsni.gov.uk) led by a Minister from the Executive. Its mission is to improve the health and social wellbeing of the people of Northern Ireland. It does this through five **NHS Health and Social Care Trusts**, which provide care locally, and the Northern Ireland Ambulance Service, which covers the whole region (www.n-i.nhs.uk).

There is a **Health and Social Care Board** which works with the Trusts to ensure services meet the needs of the population. It also commissions services through local commissioning groups and manages the financial aspects of health and social care provision (www.hscboard. hscni.net).

The **Local Commissioning Groups** are responsible for assessing health and social care needs as well as planning and securing the delivery of health and social care to meet current and emerging needs. They are sub-committees of the Health and Social Care Board and are coterminous with the five Trusts.

There is a **Public Health Agency** which is a multi-professional organisation with the mandate to protect public health, improve public health and social wellbeing and reduce inequalities in health and social wellbeing (www.publichealth.hscni.net). In addition, there is a **Patient and Client Council** (PCC) which acts as an independent voice for the people of Northern Ireland (www.n-i.nhs.uk).

The **Regulation and Quality Improvement Agency** is an independent public body, sponsored by the Department of Health, Social Services and Public Safety, which has overall responsibility for monitoring and inspecting the availability and quality of health and social care services in Northern Ireland and encouraging improvements in the quality of those services. It is accountable through the Department to the Minister.

ACTIVITY 7.4b

If you work in Northern Ireland, which of the above organisations most recently interacted with your organisation, and why?

Scotland

Following devolution and the Scotland Act in 1998, the Scottish Executive (officially referred to as the Scottish Government since August 2007) and Scottish Parliament were officially convened in 1999. This followed the transfer of powers, including those relating to health and social care services, from the Westminster Parliament (www.scotland.gov.uk). Each of the Directorates of the Scottish Government is headed by a Director-General, and the Health and Social Care Directorates are responsible for NHS Scotland as well as the development and implementation of policies relating to health and community care. Several different policies and strategies have been developed since devolution which focus specifically on the health and social care needs of the Scottish population and a number of organisations have been set up in order to develop, deliver, regulate and enhance the health and wellbeing of people in Scotland. Below are a brief description and the web addresses of some of the key organisations.

NHS Scotland, which is accountable to the Health and Social Care Directorates, has 14 Territorial NHS Health Boards and a number of **special NHS Boards**, including Healthcare Improvement Scotland and NHS Health Scotland. (www.scotland.gov.uk)

Community Health Partnerships (CHPs) provide integrated health and social care in primary and community settings under the different NHS Health Boards. There is no one model that they have to follow, so each community health partnership aligns its responsibilities to local circumstances and populations. (www.chp.scot.nhs.uk)

Healthcare Improvement Scotland (HIS) is the independent healthcare services regulator in Scotland. It has taken over the work of the Care Commission in Scotland and NHS Quality Improvement Scotland to improve the quality of the care in Scotland. It supports the delivery of Scottish Government priorities, in particular those arising from the Healthcare Quality Strategy for NHS Scotland. (www.healthcareimprovementscotland.org)

Social Care and Social Work Improvement Scotland (SCSWIS) inspects, regulates and supports the improvement of care and social work and child protection services across Scotland. It is an independent board which is partially funded by the Scottish Government.

NHS Health Scotland is the national agency for improving the health of Scotland's people. Its remit ranges from the gathering of evidence to planning, delivery and evaluation across a range of health topics, settings and life stages. (www.healthscotland.com)

The Scottish Social Services Council (SSSC) is responsible for registering people who work in social services and regulating their education and training. Its role is to raise standards of practice and increase the protection of service users and carers. (www.sssc.uk.com)

Convention of Scottish Local Authorities (COSLA) is the national voice for local government in Scotland. It enables a wide range of councillors from across the political spectrum and across Scotland to be involved in policy development to help individuals and families improve their health and wellbeing. Their health and social care team works at the interface between Scottish local government and NHS Scotland.

NHS inform is a national health information service which provides a single source of quality-assured health information for the public in Scotland (www.nhsinform.co.uk). It also has links to www.show.scot.nhs.uk, www.nhs24.com and www.keepwellscotland.org.uk.

ACTIVITY 7.4c

If you work in Scotland, which of the above organisations most recently interacted with your organisation, and why?

Wales

The Government of Wales Act 1998 established the National Assembly for Wales (www.assemblywales.org) and Welsh Assembly Government (www.wales.gov.uk) as well as reforming certain Welsh public bodies and abolishing certain others. The Welsh Assembly is made up of 60 elected members and the Welsh Government comprises 14 assembly members. There is a **Health and Social Services Directorate General** run by a director-general. He chairs a **National Delivery Group** which develops policy, plans the development and oversees delivery of NHS services.

The **National Advisory Board (NAB)** has responsibility for providing independent advice to assist the Minister in discharging her/his functions and meeting accountabilities for the performance of the NHS in Wales.

There are 22 **Local Authorities** who deliver social services and social care to the Welsh population through a number of provider organisations. The local authorities have the statutory responsibility for planning, assessment, commissioning and delivery of social services across Wales. (www.wales.gov.uk)

The seven **Local Health Boards** have a joint responsibility with local authorities to produce the local health, social care and wellbeing strategy. They are responsible for planning, designing, developing and securing the delivery of primary, community and in-hospital care services, and also, where appropriate, specialised services.

There is a **Welsh Ambulance Service NHS Trust** which provides pre-hospital emergency care and treatment throughout Wales. **Velindre NHS Trust** provides a range of cancer specialist services at local, regional and all-Wales levels. The **Public Health Wales NHS Trust** provides specialist infection and communicable disease control services.

The **Welsh Partnership Forum** is where the Welsh Government, NHS Wales employers and trade unions and professional organisations work together to improve health services for the people of Wales.

The **Care and Social Services Inspectorate Wales (CSSIW)** is the focus for professional assessment and judgement about social care, early years and social services across Wales and is responsible for ensuring an integrated approach to social services and care.

The **Social Services Improvement Agency (SSIA)** is a partnership enterprise between the Local Government Association (which hosts the SSIA), the Directors for Social Services Cymru and the Welsh Assembly Government. Its role is to support local authorities to improve service delivery and promote excellence. (www.ssiacymru.org.uk)

ACTIVITY 7.4d

If you work in Wales, which of the above organisations most recently interacted with your organisation, and why?

NON-LOCATION-SPECIFIC SERVICES

The influence of the internet

The subject of the increased expectations of service users and carers was introduced in *Chapter 1*. These expectations have been increased because of the information revolution, brought about by advancing technology and the increased access to a high level of information about health and care.

NHS Direct, the telephone information and assessment service, began in 1998 and then went online in 2008. Now, **NHS Choices: your health, your choices** is the single largest health website in the UK. It is a comprehensive information service that helps service users look after their own health care. It draws together the knowledge and expertise of NHS Evidence: Health Information Resource, the Information Centre for Health and Social Care and the Care Quality Commission, as well as several other health and social care organisations. It has over 40 interactive tools to help people self-assess and learn about their health and lifestyles. Councils are able to place a directory of local NHS and other health and social care services onto the NHS Choices website. (www.nhs.uk/aboutNHSChoices)

THE RISE IN STATUS OF THE SERVICE USER AND CARER

Over the years the terms patient, client and user have been used interchangeably; however, service user is now the term most commonly used. Service user and carer involvement has become a central theme in the agenda of successive governments. For example, it was included in *Fulfilled Lives, Supportive Communities* (Welsh Assembly Government, 2007) and *A Quality Strategy for Social Care 2000* (Department of Health, 2000a) and in many other documents before having a very strong presence in the White Paper for England, *Equity and Excellence: Liberating the NHS* (Department of Health, 2010a), which placed patients at the heart of the NHS. The Secretary of State for Health at the time regularly acknowledged his support for the service user in speeches and interviews with the media, identifying 'no decision about me, without me'.

ACTIVITY 7.5

How would you define a service user?

Warren (2007) suggests that you should answer that question by completing the statement 'I believe a service user is.........' five times, completing the sentence in a different way each time. Historically, 'service users' was the term used to describe people who were receiving services or support in order to carry out their activities of daily living. They could be mental health service users, young people being looked after in care, older people, those with physical or sensory impairment, etc.; anyone accessing health and social care services. Nowadays the term is also used to include those people who are eligible to receive their own health services (Beresford, 2000, in Warren, 2007).

ACTIVITY 7.6

How would you define a carer?

There are a wide range of people who interact with a service user who could be identified as a carer – a child, a parent, a partner or a friend. Often a service user may have several carers, who relate to them in different ways and for a greater or lesser amount of time. It is also worth remembering that the carers' interests may not always be the same as those of the service users.

ACTIVITY 7.7

What do you think the benefits are to an organisation of service user and carer involvement?

You could have given many different answers to *Activity 7.7*. However, one of the key ways in which the involvement of service users and carers adds value to an organisation is the unique perspective that they bring. No one else can have the same experience from first contact through to discharge that the service user or their carer can; it is their personal journey. Their unique body of knowledge about their own condition means that they are also experts in that condition. Whatever the reason for an individual being a service user, you will need to explore strategies to enable them to actively participate and engage with you. It is very important to have an awareness of the different perspectives of involvement because this can affect who is involved and how information is gained during the process.

ACTIVITY 7.8

How might the involvement of service users and carers help you as a leader?

The unique knowledge base that service users and carers bring to any consultation, formal or informal, can be invaluable to you in helping you to develop the services you offer. It can give you feedback on the care you are offering and the opportunities available to improve or enhance it. This feedback could also be used in order to challenge traditional assumptions about services and contribute new or innovative ideas to strategic planning. Service users and carers can help you target services better so they are more effective and give better value for money. For a leader, access to this 'insider' information is invaluable as it can add a different dimension to how you provide services to them and other service users and carers.

It is very important, however, that you use the knowledge and understanding gained in *Chapters 4* and *5* regarding culture and power to ensure that the experience for the service user is as positive for them as it is for you as a service provider. Ideally it should be a two-way relationship. A further critical point concerning service user involvement is that because of their active participation in their care, the balance of the relationship between you may shift. As an expert on their condition, they are partners in their care and may even become the leader in their care. However, it should also be noted that the concept of service users as 'customers' is emerging, which will impact on the relationship still further.

THE CHANGING LOCUS OF LEADERSHIP IN HEALTH AND SOCIAL CARE SERVICES

Throughout this book emphasis has been placed on potential for leaders to be present at all levels within an organisation. Changes in government policy over the years have led to an increasing commitment to this type of leadership by senior management and policy makers, as it is seen to strengthen an organisation and facilitate its success. With the service user becoming recognised as the 'expert' in their own condition and taking a more proactive role in managing their care, it has become increasingly important that health and care leadership is present at all levels within an organisation. In addition, with the increasing involvement of service users and carers in service development and evaluation as well as the shift in balance of power at the point of care towards the service user, the potential value of distributed leadership can be seen to be further enhanced.

CHAPTER SUMMARY

Three key points to take away from Chapter 7:

- An understanding of the structure and function of the NHS and care services, at both national and local levels, is important to you as an emerging leader as it forms the context in which you work and helps you recognise the relationships between different organisations and agencies.

- A knowledge and understanding of Government policies and their impact on your organisation is also important as it underpins both the way in which care is delivered and where it is delivered.

- Service users and carers bring a unique perspective, an understanding of which is invaluable to you as a leader due to the shift in balance in the service user–service provider relationship. With the service user becoming a leader in their own care, there is an increased need for leadership to become distributed across all levels of an organisation.

QUESTIONS

Question 7.1

Describe the structure of health and social care provision in the UK country in which you live. *(Learning outcome 7.1)*

Question 7.2

Outline the latest policy changes that have affected your workplace from both national and regional perspectives. *(Learning outcome 7.2)*

Question 7.3

Identify the ways in which the role of the service user and their carers has changed in recent years and reflect on their role in your workplace. *(Learning outcome 7.3)*

Question 7.4

Thinking about your own workplace, discuss where leadership roles are located in your organisation. *(Learning outcome 7.4)*

FURTHER READING

Horner, N. (2006) *What is Social Work? Context and Perspective*, 2nd edition. Exeter: Learning Matters.

Warren, J. (2007) *Service User and Carer Participation in Social Work*. Exeter: Learning Matters.

www.nhshistory.net

Because of the pace of change in the health and social care sector, it is advisable for you to look at key websites rather than rely on books or journal articles in relation to the up-to-date structure and function of the NHS and social care services.

8

LEADERSHIP DEVELOPMENT – SO WHERE DO YOU GO FROM HERE?

LEARNING OUTCOMES:

When you have completed this chapter you should be able to:

8.1 Discuss the role of reflective practice in leadership development

8.2 Identify your leadership development objectives

8.3 Outline your current strengths and weaknesses as a leader and the threats and opportunities that may impact on your leadership development

8.4 Identify opportunities for experiential learning in your leadership development

8.5 Develop an action plan which addresses your leadership development needs.

INTRODUCTION

This book has examined leadership from many different perspectives. It began by clarifying what we mean by leadership. It then went on to provide an overview of the theories of leadership, the skills and qualities of effective leaders, leadership values and culture. Power and influence have been debated and change management theory has been discussed and applied. Finally, the discussions were brought together in the context of the leadership agenda in health and social care today.

You have therefore read a great deal and engaged in activities concerned with many of the facets of leadership. This alone, however, will not enable you to achieve your potential as a leader. There is no magic wand that will transform you overnight into the kind of leader you want to be. Leadership development is a conscious process that requires a reflective approach to practice.

This final chapter aims to support you in truly unleashing your potential as a leader. It addresses practical strategies that you can use as part of your personal and professional development to further develop yourself as a leader.

WHERE ARE YOU NOW?

In order to develop yourself as a leader you need to accurately assess both your capabilities and learning needs throughout your lifetime as a leader. As outlined in *Chapter 3*, self-awareness is pivotal in refining and developing leadership performance. One method of enhancing self-awareness and clarifying where you are now in your leadership capabilities is through reflection. There are various approaches to enhancing one's ability to reflect on practice.

What is reflection and reflective practice?

SCENARIO 8.1

Julie was new in post as a specialist nurse. She was experienced clinically in her area of practice but was inexperienced as a leader. Julie was asked to lead a project which involved recruitment of staff and leadership of them to safely set up a new service. Julie got on with the job to the best of her ability; however, when the records of the selection interviews were reviewed by the Personnel department, it was found that Julie had not adhered to the Trust's recruitment and selection policy. Personnel advised Julie that she should have undertaken training with them before undertaking recruitment and selection. All candidates therefore had to be re-interviewed, although Julie had already told several that they had been selected for the post.

Julie felt that she had fallen at the first hurdle. She was very embarrassed. On reflecting on the situation she recognised that she had been so anxious to prove herself that she had blindly got on with the job, rather than recognising where she needed support and using the support networks available in the Trust. The Director of Personnel also reflected on the experience and realised that recruitment and selection procedures had been overlooked in the Trust's induction programme. The programme was therefore altered accordingly.

This scenario illustrates how reflection can help make sense of situations and enhance self-awareness. Johns (2002) describes reflection as a process which enables individuals to develop an understanding of how and why situations and events have occurred. If done well, it has the potential to be transformational in terms of helping people to change in themselves as well as in relation to their practice (Ghaye & Lillyman, 2000).

Reflective practice enables the practitioner to integrate theory with practice through consciously thinking through events (Jasper, 2003). The conscious process of applying knowledge to the situation may occur during the incident itself (reflection-in-action) or after the event (reflection-on-action) (Schön, 1991).

You may reflect already; many of us do. However, there are varying layers of reflection, ranging from 'doing reflection' to reflection being an integral part of your daily practice (Johns, 2004). The different layers of reflection are summarised in *Figure 8.1*.

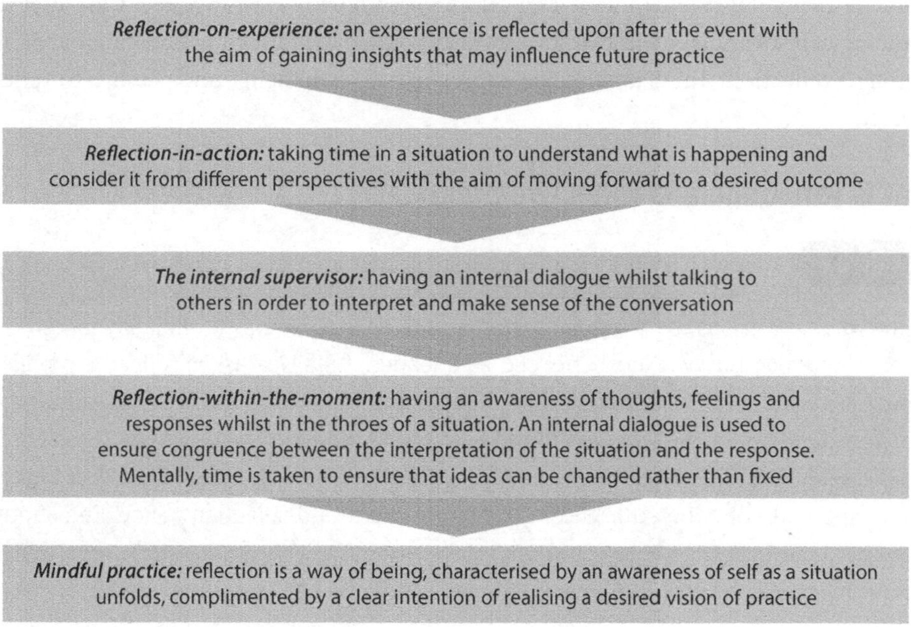

Reflection-on-experience: an experience is reflected upon after the event with the aim of gaining insights that may influence future practice

Reflection-in-action: taking time in a situation to understand what is happening and consider it from different perspectives with the aim of moving forward to a desired outcome

The internal supervisor: having an internal dialogue whilst talking to others in order to interpret and make sense of the conversation

Reflection-within-the-moment: having an awareness of thoughts, feelings and responses whilst in the throes of a situation. An internal dialogue is used to ensure congruence between the interpretation of the situation and the response. Mentally, time is taken to ensure that ideas can be changed rather than fixed

Mindful practice: reflection is a way of being, characterised by an awareness of self as a situation unfolds, complimented by a clear intention of realising a desired vision of practice

Figure 8.1 *Layers of reflection (adapted from Johns, 2004)*

To aid the reflective process a number of different reflective models and cycles have been developed.

Reflective models

Reflective models can act as a guide to help you structure your reflections and identify the various aspects of your learning through reflection (Howatson-Jones, 2010). A particularly well-known and popular model is Johns' model for structured reflection (Johns, 2004). The model uses a sequential list of cues that aim to facilitate the individual in reflecting deeply and broadly to maximise their learning through experience. The cues are detailed in *Figure 8.2*.

⇨ Bring the mind home – give myself the space and time to reflect through relaxing and clearing the mind

⇨ Describe the experience

⇨ Identify the issues that seem most significant

⇨ How did others feel and why did they feel like this?

⇨ How did I feel and what made me feel like that?

⇨ What was I aiming to achieve and did I respond appropriately?

⇨ What were the outcomes of my actions on others and me?

⇨ What factors influence my thoughts, feelings or responses?

⇨ What knowledge informed me or could have informed me?

⇨ To what degree did I adhere to my values and act for the best?

⇨ How do previous experiences connect with this situation?

⇨ How could I respond more effectively if the situation arose again?

⇨ What would the consequences of alternative actions be for me and others?

⇨ How do I feel about the experience now?

⇨ Am I now more able to support myself and others as a result of the experience?

⇨ Am I able to achieve desirable practice using appropriate frameworks?

Figure 8.2 *Model for structured reflection – the reflective cues (adapted from Johns, 2004)*

ACTIVITY 8.1

Identify a leadership situation that you have been a part of and use Johns' model for structured reflection (Johns, 2004) to reflect on and learn from the situation.

You may also wish to explore Atkins and Murphy's (1995) model of reflection which identifies three stages of reflection. Stage 1 is concerned with the awareness of uncomfortable feelings which may be associated with a new situation or a challenge. Stage 2 focuses on a critical analysis of the situation where feelings are related to knowledge through examining the impact of knowledge or deficits in knowledge on the situation and the effects of the individual on the experience. Stage 3 aims to help the learner develop new perspectives on the experience and to identify how they will apply their learning to future experiences.

ACTIVITY 8.2

Apply Atkins and Murphy's (1995) model of reflection to another leadership situation that you have been a part of. Which model suits you best? Did you feel that both models could be used together?

Many reflective models exist and it would be in your interests to use the recommended reading at the end of this chapter to explore further models. Your choice of model should be guided by personal preference and it may be that you find a combination of models of use, for example Johns' (2004) cues may have helped you to apply Atkins and Murphy's (1995) model more comprehensively.

Reflective cycles

Reflective cycles aim to enable the individual to link what they have learned from previous experiences to new experiences. Gibbs' reflective cycle is one of the most well known of these cycles (Gibbs, 1988) and lends itself well to leadership development due to the action planning element which helps the individual focus on how their analysis can be taken forward. Gibbs' reflective cycle is summarised in *Figure 8.3*.

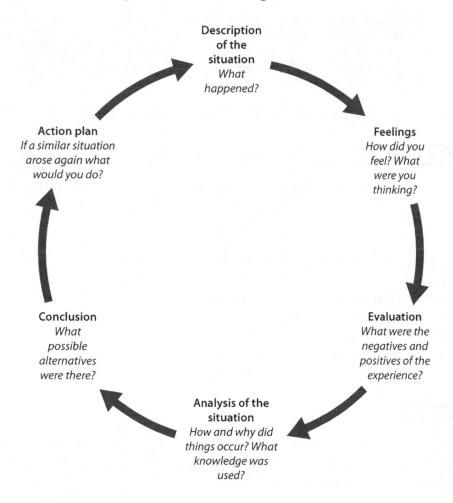

Figure 8.3 *Gibbs' reflective cycle (adapted from Gibbs, 1988)*

ACTIVITY 8.3

Return to Julie's scenario (*Scenario 8.1*). How could Julie apply Gibbs' reflective cycle (Gibbs, 1988)?

STRENGTHS, WEAKNESSES, OPPORTUNITIES AND THREATS

A SWOT analysis can be of great use in assessing where you are at any point in time with regard to your leadership development and how you can take your development forward. SWOT is an acronym for:

Strengths

Weaknesses

Opportunities

Threats

Strengths will vary from one individual to the next. They may include qualities that are innate or acquired through practice. Examples may include aspects of your communication skills such as an ability to communicate your thoughts clearly, eye contact or assertiveness. Other skills and qualities may relate to your effect on others, for example an ability to motivate, emotional intelligence and a positive disposition. Others may be related to your ability to accomplish tasks, such as your ability to learn quickly, flexibility and open-mindedness.

Weaknesses are areas that require further development. Again, these will be unique to the individual and will encompass aspects of your leadership performance that concern your ability to relate to others and to fulfil specific tasks. At this stage in your development, these may include a lack of knowledge and experience of the field of work or a lack of experience of using different leadership styles. Such limitations may then impact on other areas of your performance such as your ability to be flexible and adaptable.

Opportunities relate to any potential openings for you to utilise in order to further develop your leadership skills. These may include, for example, the use of role models, coaching, mentoring and 360° feedback. These will be discussed later in this chapter.

Threats are concerned with potential barriers to your development. Issues may relate to the availability of resources, culture of the organisation or issues that are personal to you. Examples of the latter may include a lack of self-belief, confidence or motivation.

ACTIVITY 8.4

Complete a SWOT analysis of your current leadership abilities using the grid below. You may find it useful to use a mind map as a way of identifying each of these areas (see p. 29).

STRENGTHS	WEAKNESSES
OPPORTUNITIES	THREATS

The potential of a SWOT analysis for leadership development depends upon taking the analysis further. Once the strengtchs, weaknesses, opportunities and threats have been identified, thought needs to be given to how strengths and opportunities can be maximised and how weaknesses and threats can be minimised. Strengths-based leadership theory suggests that energy should be focused on the further development of your leadership strengths and on exploiting opportunities to further develop these. Through doing this it is argued that weaknesses and threats will naturally be minimised (Rath & Conchie, 2008).

An additional way of fully utilising a SWOT analysis is through action planning which will now be explored.

WHERE DO YOU WANT TO BE?

An essential aspect of leadership development is underpinned by having a vision of what you wish to accomplish as a leader. Through having a clear vision you can form a plan that you can work towards on a daily basis to ensure that your vision is realised.

ACTIVITY 8.5

Draw a mind map of all that you hope to achieve as a leader. After doing this, have a break and then return to your mind map. Try to form a statement that captures all that you wish to achieve as a leader. This is called a vision statement.

Depending upon where you are in your leadership journey, your vision may focus on your own personal development or perhaps be more complex, relating to the accomplishment of a specific goal through your team. Vision statements from a range of health and social care students are given in *Figure 8.4*.

Once you have identified your vision the next step is to identify how you are going to realise your goal. The vision statement can be viewed as your overarching aim and the next step is to identify the objectives that will enable you to achieve your vision. Objectives need to be SMART:

Specific

Measurable

Attainable

Relevant

Timebound

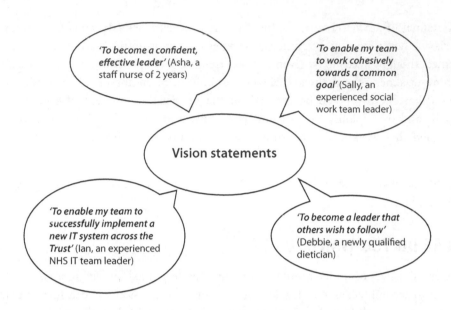

Figure 8.4 *Vision statements*

ACTIVITY 8.6

Return to your SWOT analysis and vision statement. Identify what you need to do in order to achieve your vision. State what you need to have as SMART objectives.

People across all professions consistently find it difficult to set SMART objectives. The following scenarios will help you decide whether your objectives are clearly expressed.

Debbie's leadership vision is *'to become a leader that others wish to follow'*. In order to achieve this Debbie has identified four objectives that she aims to achieve within the next 12 months:

- To be able to communicate assertively when required

- To be perceived as a leader

- To develop negotiation skills

- To develop a range of leadership styles.

SCENARIO 8.2

Debbie qualified and got her first post as a dietician six months ago. She has lots of new ideas about how the Trust's dietetic services could be enhanced. However, Debbie is nervous about expressing her ideas for change as she feels that she has little influence amongst her more experienced colleagues due to her newly qualified status. Debbie is also naturally quiet and finds it difficult to challenge others and communicate assertively. Her SWOT analysis of her leadership performance is as follows:

STRENGTHS	WEAKNESSES
• Emotionally intelligent • Able to adapt to change • Very quick learner • Knowledgeable • Stimulated by new ideas	• Inexperienced • Finds it difficult to voice opinion • Lacking in assertiveness • Unwilling to lead • Does not like to challenge others
OPPORTUNITIES	THREATS
• In-house education • Role modelling • Networking • Coaching • Mentoring	• Lack of a coach or mentor • Lack of formal educational support • Low confidence • A lack of self-belief

ACTIVITY 8.7

What actions could Debbie take in order to achieve these objectives?

In order to achieve her first objective, Debbie could access an assertiveness training course through the Trust's in-house educational programme, she could seek out a coach and she could practise being assertive in non-threatening situations. She needs to do all of this within the next six months.

To achieve her second objective, Debbie needs to focus on how she communicates and behaves. To help with this she may need to reflect regularly using a reflective model such as Johns' (2004) and she may wish to utilise the Trust's clinical supervision programme. She may also wish to make use of a mentor. Debbie will be able to commence these actions promptly and continue with them throughout the 12-month timeframe.

Achievement of her third objective will be underpinned by achievement of Debbie's first objective and also by Debbie familiarising herself with principled negotiation techniques (see p. 90) and practising these. Because of the interdependence with the first objective, Debbie will need to embark on developing her skills in principled negotiation in six months' time.

The final objective could be achieved through Debbie accessing a course of study, reading leadership articles and texts, utilising action learning sets and practising adapting her leadership style to different contexts and situations. Debbie should aim to achieve all of this within nine months.

Coaching, clinical supervision and action learning sets are discussed below, along with other leadership development opportunities, which you will find of value in your journey to fully realising your potential as a leader.

CLINICAL SUPERVISION

Clinical supervision is also known as 'practice support'. This term is often used as an alternative, to get away from the notion of this style of support being applicable only to those working in clinical environments and also from the supervisory suggestion of the title (Lillyman, 2007a). Practice support is a formal, yet voluntary process. It is flexible in its approach, depending upon the learning styles of the individual(s) and usually takes place on a one-to-one, group or networking basis every four to six weeks at a pre-arranged time. Meetings can last from one to two hours, depending upon the size and availability of the group. Discussions involve reflecting on practice in order to learn from practice and enhance performance (King's Fund, 1995). The *one-to-one* approach consists of a supervisor and a supervisee. The supervisor may be a peer or someone with expertise in the field who can guide the supervisee in the areas that they raise. *Group supervision* usually includes up to six members who have a common interest. For example, a group may consist of leaders who are employed across a range of health and social care services, or a group may consist of staff from a particular area of work, for example a team of speech and language therapists specialising in stroke rehabilitation. A supervisor normally guides the discussions and reflections, although this role may be rotated within the group. The *networking* approach is suitable for those who work in isolated areas, such as specialist posts, where group members may seek out individuals employed in similar roles outside the immediate workplace (Lillyman, 2007a).

Debbie (*Scenario 8.2*) is likely to find one-to-one or group clinical supervision of use in addressing her second objective '*to be perceived as a leader*'. Sessions could be used to help her to reflect upon how she conveys herself and to build her confidence.

ACTION LEARNING SETS

Action learning is based on the argument that learning does not take place without action and that no thoughtful, purposeful action occurs without learning (Pedler, 1997). Action learning sets offer a framework for promoting this process and have been used in management and leadership since the 1970s (Lillyman, 2007b).

The set (or group) is made up of 6 to 8 professionals who may be peers (for example a set of matrons), or may work in different contexts across different levels within the organisation (for example a multi-professional group with a common interest in end of life care). The group meet at regular intervals in an environment away from work where people feel safe to speak openly. A facilitator assists the group to listen, question and challenge individuals, which culminates in the individual developing an action plan aimed at addressing the issue reflected upon.

The meeting starts with an individual volunteering to share their issue or concern with the group. They tell their story without interruption. Once the story has been told, the group and facilitator may ask questions to seek clarification and to summarise the points made. Once the story is clear to the group, members can then ask open, challenging questions, but at no point should advice or opinions be offered. The rationale for this is that it allows the presenter to explore the issues for him- or herself and therefore promotes a deeper level of reflection. Questions aim to assist reflection and help the presenter move forward through the development of an action plan, but care must be taken that through being challenged the presenter is not made to feel distressed. The presenter is given time to critically reflect, to give feedback to the group and to formulate a plan of action (Lillyman, 2007b).

Following implementation of the action plan, the individual reports their progress to the group at the beginning of the next meeting. Progress may be positive, in which case another issue may be reflected upon or implementation may not have been achieved, in which case the issues are explored further through listening, questioning and challenging and a further action plan is developed.

Debbie (*Scenario 8.2*) is going to use action learning sets as a way of helping her *'to develop a range of leadership styles'* (her fourth objective). Action learning sets have been used successfully by the author in helping leaders apply leadership theory to practice, following engagement with leadership development programmes. The process enables the individual to shift the focus from thought to action through applying and further developing their learning (Lillyman, 2007b).

COACHING

Debbie (*Scenario 8.2*) is going to use coaching to help her develop her assertiveness skills. Debbie is naturally quiet and finds it difficult to challenge others and communicate assertively.

ACTIVITY 8.8

What does coaching mean to you? What are its aims? How does it differ from clinical supervision and action learning sets?

Coaching is concerned with facilitating the performance, learning and development of an individual. It aims to shift the focus from the problem to goal-orientated behaviour. Coaching usually takes place in a one-to-one context at a pre-arranged time and place. However, coaching can become part of a leader's toolkit and can be used as and when required. It is also sometimes used to facilitate the performance and development of a group.

There are many different approaches to coaching, ranging from non-directive (where the coach listens, reflects, paraphrases, summarises and asks awareness-raising questions) to highly directive, where the coach may offer suggestions, offer guidance, give advice or instruct (Downey, 2003). The approach will be determined by the learning style of the person being coached. Discussions are focused and purposeful, with an emphasis on encouragement, strengths and solutions. Coaching aims to enhance self-awareness and uses everyday work as a learning experience. It is a non-hierarchical process.

Alexander and Renshaw (2005) emphasise the importance of coaching qualities. These focus on three areas which are interdependent: the relationship, being and doing. The relationship is concerned with values, honesty and openness, the ability to be supportive yet challenging and organisational awareness. Being is characterised by self-awareness, enabling and self-confidence. Doing encompasses a clear methodology, accomplished skills in communication and the use of an enabling framework (Alexander & Renshaw, 2005).

The GROW model (Whitmore, 2002) is a widely used coaching model. It provides a framework for a coaching session encompassing four key elements which are referred to using the acronym 'GROW':

Goal

Reality

Options

Will

Every coaching session has a specific Goal. The Goal is established at the beginning of the session. It should be measurable so that its achievement is clear. An appropriate Goal for one of Debbie's coaching sessions may be that she develops strategies to help her communicate assertively when she needs to. Once the Goal is clear, the GROW model advocates that the coaching session goes on to help the individual explore the current Reality; in other words, where they are starting from. This aims to help the individual see the situation clearly and is often of great value in helping the individual identify the way forward. Next, Options are explored that will help the individual achieve their Goal. In Debbie's scenario, options may include practical strategies for assertive communication or overcoming psychological barriers. Finally the session closes with a commitment to action, which the GROW model calls Will. This may include action planning, consideration of any implications and obstacles, identification of support and reference to the original goal.

Other coaching models that you may wish to explore are STEPPA and the Conscious Competence Model.

360° FEEDBACK

As you progress through your leadership career, self-awareness remains just as important as it is at your current stage. 360° feedback is an additional method of enhancing this awareness and reducing the 'blind spot' described in *Chapter 3* in relation to the Johari window (*Figure 3.4*). It aims to help you gain an insight into how others perceive and interpret your leadership behaviours.

360° feedback and the 360° feedback process involve the collection of information regarding the performance of an individual. Feedback is sought from a variety of sources such as peers, managers, staff who work for the individual, clients or patients and the individual him- or herself. The information is then compiled by a trained facilitator to form a report that is given to the individual. The 360° feedback process provides further input by providing appropriate follow-up training and support. Information is then sought again from colleagues, clients or patients and the individual, and the data are compiled into a report for presentation to the individual (Shipper *et al.*, 2007).

The feedback document is a questionnaire which is designed around the key skill areas of the individual's roles. These are broken down into elements and measured by carefully worded questions, which the respondents answer and rank the individual's performance. Some areas of health and social care have pre-designed questionnaires which reflect the objectives of the organisation. For example, the 'NHS 360° Feedback Tool' is aligned with the NHS Leadership Qualities Framework discussed in *Chapter 3* (NHS Institute for Innovation and Improvement, 2009).

ACTIVITY 8.9

Make a list of the key skill areas that underpin your role as a leader. What aspects of your role would you appreciate feedback on? Who could you ask for their opinions?

360° feedback has become a largely commercialised venture but there is still value in seeking out others' opinions yourself. It is worth noting, however, that the value of 360° feedback across cultures has been questioned (Shipper *et al.*, 2007). Also, some people lack skill in giving feedback in a constructive manner. It is therefore advised that you carry out your own 360° feedback with the support of a trained facilitator.

LEARNING FROM DOING

This book has offered you a great deal of practical advice underpinned by theoretical perspectives. By helping you to become more self-aware and more knowledgeable it can help you learn and become a more effective leader. If you apply all that you have learnt you will hold great promise. However, no one can make you an effective leader but yourself. Reading a book on mountaineering will not make you a great mountaineer and reading a book about athletics will not make you an Olympic athlete. Leadership is no different! It is only through applying all that you have read and learnt that you will unleash your potential as a leader.

DEVELOPING AN ACTION PLAN

This chapter therefore ends with a final task:

ACTIVITY 8.10

Identify the actions that you need to take in order to achieve your leadership vision in the form of an action plan, as detailed below:

Your vision statement:

Your objectives (informed by your vision, your reflections, feedback from colleagues and your SWOT analysis):

Your Action Plan:

Objective	*Actions to be taken*	*Date*

Make sure that you do as you plan and enjoy the journey!

CHAPTER SUMMARY

Three key points to take away from Chapter 8:

- In order to develop as a leader, a heightened self-awareness is required. This can be facilitated through reflection, clinical supervision, action learning sets, coaching and peer review.

- The development of leadership skills and qualities can be enhanced through systematically identifying learning needs and planning how these will be met. Action planning is one approach to facilitating this process.

- Your development as a leader will be a never-ending journey – enjoy it and look after yourself on the way!

QUESTIONS

Question 8.1

Which model of reflection would best facilitate you in your development as a leader? *(Learning outcome 8.1)*

Question 8.2

List four objectives which will support your development as a leader. *(Learning outcome 8.2)*

Question 8.3

How does your SWOT analysis relate to your leadership development objectives? *(Learning outcome 8.3)*

Question 8.4

How do you access clinical supervision, action learning sets and coaching in your place of work? *(Learning outcome 8.4)*

Question 8.5

Make a list of colleagues and services available to you at work that will help you in implementing your action plan. *(Learning outcome 8.5)*

FURTHER READING

Howatson-Jones, L. (2010) *Reflective Practice in Nursing.* Exeter: Learning Matters.

Johns, C. (2004) *Becoming a Reflective Practitioner*, 2nd edition. Oxford: Blackwell Publishing.

Lillyman, S. & Ghaye, T. (2007) *Effective Clinical Supervision: The Role of Reflection*, 2nd edition. London: Quay Books.

REFERENCES

Adair, J. (2009) *Not Bosses But Leaders. How to Lead the Way to Success*, 3rd edition. London: Kogan Page.

Akerjordet, K. & Severinsson, E. (2004) Emotional intelligence in mental health nurses talking about practice. *International Journal of Mental Health Nursing*, **13:** 164–170.

Alexander, G. & Renshaw, B. (2005) *Supercoaching*. London: Random House Business Books.

Alliance for Servant Leadership (2010) *Guiding Principles*. Available at www.indstate.edu/asl/principles.htm (accessed 26 April 2012)

Appleby, J. (2005) *Independent Review of Health and Social Services Care in Northern Ireland*. Available at www.dhsspsni.gov.uk/show_publications?txtid=13662 (accessed 26 April 2012)

Atkins, S. & Murphy, K. (1995) Reflective practice. *Nursing Standard*, **9(45):** 31–7.

Bandura, A. (1995) *Self-efficacy in Changing Societies*. Cambridge: Cambridge University Press.

Baron, R.A. & Greenberg, J. (1990) *Behavior in Organizations*, 3rd edition. Boston: Allyn & Bacon.

Barr, J. & Dowding, L. (2008) *Leadership in Health Care*. London: Sage.

Bass, B.M. (1985) *Leadership and Performance Beyond Expectations*. New York: Free Press.

Bass, B.M. (1990) From transactional to transformational leadership: learning to share the vision. *Organisational Dynamics*, **18(3):** 19–31.

Beckhard, R. & Harris, R. (1987) *Organizational Transitions: Managing Complex Change*, 2nd edition. Boston: Addison-Wesley.

Beecham, J. (2006) *Beyond Boundaries: Citizen-centred Local Services for Wales*. Cardiff: Welsh Assembly Government.

Bennis, W. & Nanus, B. (1985) *Leaders: The Strategies for Taking Charge*. New York: Harper & Row.

Beresford, P. (2000) Service users' knowledges and social work theory: conflict or collaboration. In: Warren, J. (2007) *Service User and Carer Participation in Social Work*. Exeter: Learning Matters.

Berne, E. (1964) *Games People Play*. Harmondsworth: Penguin.

Bernhard, L. & Walsh, M. (2006) *Leadership: The Key to Professionalization of Nursing.* St Louis: Mosby.

Bicheno , J. (2006) *The New Lean Toolbox.* Buckingham: PICSIE.

Birrell, D. (2007) *Devolution and Social Care: Are There Four Systems of Social Care in the United Kingdom?* Available at www.sochealth.co.uk/news/birrell.htm (accessed 26 April 2012)

Blake, R.R. & Mouton, J.S. (1964) *The Managerial Grid.* Houston: Gulf Publishing Co.

Block, P. (1987) *The Empowered Manager.* San Francisco: Jossey-Bass.

Brooks, I. (2009) *Organisational Behaviour: Individuals, Groups and Organisation,* 4th edition. Harlow: Prentice Hall.

Brooks, I. & Bate, P. (1994) The problems of effecting change within the British Civil Service: A cultural perspective. *British Journal of Management,* **5:** 177–190.

Burns, J.M. (1978) *Leadership.* New York: Harper & Row.

Calabria, D.C. (1982) CEOs and the paradox of power. *Business Horizons,* **25(1):** 29–31.

Chambers, R., Mohanna, K., Spurgeon, P. & Wall, D. (2007) *How to Succeed as a Leader.* Oxford: Radcliffe Publishing.

Conger, J.A. & Kanungo, R.N. (1988) The empower process: integrating theory and practice. *Academy of Management Review,* **13:** 471–482.

Cummings, G., Hayduk, L. & Estabrooks, C. (2005) Mitigating the impact of hospital restructuring on nurses. The responsibility of emotionally intelligent leadership. *Nursing Research,* **54(1):** 2–12.

Cummings, T.G. & Worley, C.G. (2005) *Organisation Development and Change,* 8th edition. Ohio: Thomson South-Western.

Daft, R.L. (1983) *Organization Theory and Design.* West Publishing Co.

Daft, R.L. (2005) *The Leadership Experience,* 3rd edition. Ohio: Thomson South-Western.

Deal, T. & Kennedy, A. (1982) *Corporate Cultures: The Rites and Rituals of Corporate Life.* Reading, MA: Addison-Wesley.

Department of the Environment, Transport and the Regions (1998) *Modern Local Government: In Touch with the People.* London: HMSO.

Department of Health (1992) *Health of the Nation.* London: HMSO.

Department of Health (1997) *The New NHS: Modern, Dependable.* London: DoH.

Department of Health (1998) *Modernising social services, promoting independence, improving protection, raising standards.* London: DoH.

Department of Health (2000a) *A quality strategy for social care 2000.* London: HMSO. Available at www.dh.gov.uk/en/Publicationsandstatistics/Publications/PublicationsPolicyAndGuidance/DH_4009379 (accessed 26 April 2012)

Department of Health (2000b) *The NHS Plan: a plan for investment, a plan for reform.* London: HMSO. Available at www.dh.gov.uk/en/Publicationsandstatistics/Publications/PublicationsPolicyandGuidance/DH_4002960 (accessed 26 April 2012)

Department of Health (2002) *Securing our Future Health: Taking a long-term view – the Wanless report.* London: HM Treasury. Available at http://www.dh.gov.uk/en/

Publicationsandstatistics/Publications/PublicationsPolicyAndGuidance/DH_4009293 (accessed 26 April 2012)

Department of Health *(*2003a) *The NHS Knowledge and Skills Framework (NHS KSF) and the Development Review Process.* London: DoH.

Department of Health (2003b) Discharge from hospital: pathway, process and practice. London: DoH.

Department of Health *(*2004) *Achieving Timely 'Simple' Discharge from Hospital. A Toolkit for the Multi-disciplinary Team.* London: DoH.

Department of Health (2007) *Our NHS Our Future: NHS Next Stage Review.* London: DoH.

Department of Health (2008) *High quality care for all: NHS Next Stage Review final report.* London: DoH. Available at www.dh.gov.uk/en/publicationsandstatistics/publications/ publicationspolicyandguidance/DH_085825 (accessed 26 April 2012)

Department of Health (2010a) *Equity and Excellence: Liberating the NHS.* White Paper, available at www.dh.gov.uk/en/Publicationsandstatistics/Publications/ PublicationsPolicyAndGuidance/DH_117353 (accessed 26 April 2012)

Department of Health (2010b) *Ready to go? Planning the discharge and the transfer of patients from hospital and intermediate care.* London: DoH. Available at www.dh.gov.uk/en/ Publicationsandstatistics/Publications/PublicationsPolicyAndGuidance/DH_113950 (accessed 26 April 2012)

Department of Health, Social Services and Public Safety (2002) *Investing for Health Strategy Review.* Available at www.dhsspsni.gov.uk/health_development-final_report_-_ september_2010.pdf (accessed 26 April 2012)

Department of Health, Social Services and Public Safety (2009) Health and Social Care (Reform) Act (Northern Ireland) 2009 (Ch. 1). Available at www.legislation.gov.uk/ nia/2009/1/pdfs/nia_20090001_en.pdf (accessed 26 April 2012)

Department of Health, Social Services and Public Safety (2011) *Transforming Your Care: A Review of Health and Social Care in Northern Ireland.* Available at www.dhsspsni.gov. uk/transforming-your-care-review-of-hsc-ni-final-report.pdf (accessed 26 April 2012)

Dowling, G. (1993) Developing your company image into a corporate asset. In: Hatch, M.J. & Schultz, M. (1997) Relations between Organizational Culture, Identity and image. *European Journal of Marketing,* **31(5/6):** 356–365. Available at fcis.vdu.lt/~n. klebanskaja@evf.vdu.lt/FOV1-00088D33/0070310502.pdf (accessed 26 April 2012)

Downey, M. (2003) *Effective Coaching: Lessons from the Coach's Coach.* Los Angeles: Texere Publishing.

Downton, J.V. (1973) *Rebel Leadership: Commitment and Charisma in a Revolutionary Process.* New York: Free Press.

Eagly, A.H. (2005) Achieving relational authenticity in leadership: Does gender matter? *Leadership Quarterly,* **16:** 459–474.

Firth, K. (2002) Ward leadership: balancing the clinical and managerial roles. *Professional Nurse,* **17(8):** 486–489.

Fisher, R. & Ury, W. (1981) *Getting to Yes. Negotiating Agreement Without Giving In.* London: Hutchinson Business.

French Jr, J.R.P. & Raven, B. (1959) The bases of social power. In: Brooks, I. (2009) *Organisational Behaviour: Individuals, Groups and Organisation*, 4th edition. Harlow: Prentice Hall.

French, W. L. & Bell, C.H. (1990) *Organization Development: Behavioural Science Interventions for Organization Improvement*, 4th edition. Harlow: Prentice Hall.

Freshwater, D., Graham, I. and Esterhuizen, P. (2009) Educating leaders for global health care. In: Bishop, V. (2009) *Leadership for Nursing and Allied Health Care Professions.* Berkshire: Open University Press.

Gabbott, M. & Hogg, G. (2001) The role of non-verbal communication in service encounters: A conceptual framework. *Journal of Marketing Management,* **17(1–2):** 5–26.

Gerzon, M. (2006) *Leading Through Conflict. How Successful Leaders Transform Differences into Opportunities.* Boston: Harvard Business School Press.

Ghaye, T. & Lillyman, S. (2000) *Reflection: Principles and Practice for Healthcare Professionals.* Dinton: Quay Books / Mark Allen.

Gibbs, G. (1988) *Learning by Doing: A Guide to Teaching and Learning Methods.* Oxford: Further Education Unit, Oxford Polytechnic.

Goffee, R. & Jones, G. (2000) Why should anyone be led by you? *Harvard Business Review,* **78(5):** 62–70.

Goffee, R. & Jones, G. (2009) Authentic leadership. Excite others to exceptional performance. *Leadership Excellence,* **26(7):** 17.

Goleman, D. (1995) *Emotional Intelligence: Why it can matter more than IQ.* New York: Bantam Books.

Goleman, D. (1998a) What makes a leader? *Harvard Business Review,* **76(6):** 93–102.

Goleman, D. (1998b) *Working with Emotional Intelligence.* London: Bloomsbury.

Goleman, D. (2000) Leadership that gets results. *Harvard Business Review,* **72(2):** 78–90.

Goleman, D., Boyatzis, R.E. & McKee, A. (2009) Primal Leadership: Prime good feelings in followers. *Leadership Excellence,* **Oct:** 9–10.

Gopee, N. & Galloway, J. (2009) *Leadership and Management in Healthcare.* London: Sage.

Greenleaf, R.K. (1970) *The Servant as Leader.* Cited by: The Greenleaf Center for Servant Leadership. Available at www.greenleaf.org/whatissl/ (accessed 26 April 2012)

Handy, C.B. (1985) *Understanding Organisations*, 3rd edition. London: Penguin Business.

Hersey, P., Blanchard, K.H. & Johnson, D.E. (1996) *Management and Organizational Behavior: Utilizing Human Resources*, 7th edition. London: Prentice Hall.

Herzberg, F. (1968) *Work and the Nature of Man.* London: Crosby Lockwood Staples.

Hicks, H.G. & Gullett, C.R. (1975) *Organizations: Theory and Behavior.* New York: McGraw-Hill Book Company.

HMSO (1948) National Assistance Act (11 & 12 Geo. 6. Ch. 29). London: HMSO.

HMSO (1968) Health Services and Public Health Act (Ch. 46). London: HMSO.

HMSO (1989) Children Act (Ch. 41). London: HMSO.

HMSO (1990) *National Health Service and Community Care Act* (Ch. 19). London: HMSO.

HMSO (1999) *Local Government Act* (Ch. 27). London: HMSO.

Hofstede, G. (1984) *Culture's Consequences: International Differences in Work-related Values.* Beverly Hills, CA: Sage.

Hofstede, G. (1991) *Cultures and Organizations.* Maidenhead: McGraw-Hill.

Hofstede, G. (2001) *Culture's Consequences: Comparing Values, Behaviors, Institutions, and Organizations Across Nations.* Thousand Oaks, CA: Sage.

Hofstede, G. & Hofstede G.J. (2005) *Cultures and Organizations: Software of the Mind*, 2nd edition. New York: McGraw Hill.

Honey, P. & Mumford, A. (1986) *Using Your Learning Style.* Maidenhead: Peter Honey Publications.

Horner, N. (2006) *What is Social Work? Context and Perspectives*, 2nd edition. Exeter: Learning Matters.

Howatson-Jones, I.L. (2004) The servant leader. *Nursing Management,* **11(3):** 20–24.

Howatson-Jones, L. (2010) *Reflective Practice in Nursing.* Exeter: Learning Matters Ltd.

Huber, D. (2010) *Leadership and Nursing Care Management*, 4th edition. Missouri: Saunders Elsevier.

Iles, V. (2006) *Really Managing Health Care*, 2nd edition. Berkshire: Open University Press.

Illumine (2010) *How to Make a Mind Map.* Available at www.mind-mapping.co.uk/make-mind-map.htm (accessed 26 April 2012)

Jasper, M. (2003) *Beginning Reflective Practice.* Cheltenham:Nelson Thornes.

Jervis, P. & Plowden, W. (2003) *The Impact of Political Devolution on the UK Health Services.* London: The Nuffield Trust.

Johns, C. (2002) *Guided Reflection: Advancing Practice.* Oxford: Blackwell Science.

Johns, C. (2004) *Becoming a Reflective Practitioner*, 2nd edition. Oxford: Blackwell Publishing.

Johnson, G. & Scholes, K. (2005) *Exploring Corporate Strategy*, 8th edition. Harlow: Financial Times Prentice Hall.

Jones, R. & Jenkins, F. (2006) *Managing and Leading in the Allied Health Professions.* Oxford: Radcliffe Publishing.

Kanter, R.M. (1983) *The Change Masters.* Simon & Schuster: New York.

Katz, R.L. (1955) Skills of an effective administrator. *Harvard Business Review,* **33(1):** 33–42.

Kilmann, R. (2010) *The Thomas–Kilmann Conflict Mode Instrument. Available at* http://kilmann.com/conflict.html (accessed 26 April 2012)

King's Fund (1995) *Clinical Supervision: An Executive Summary.* London: King's Fund.

Kotter, J.P. (1985) *Power and Influence: Beyond Formal Authority.* New York: Free Press.

Kotter, J.P. (1996) *Leading Change.* Boston: Harvard Business School Press.

Kubler-Ross, E. (1973) *On Death and Dying.* London: Routledge.

Lewin, K. (1947) Frontiers in group dynamics: Concept, method and reality in social science; social equilibria and social change. *Human Relations,* **1:** 5–41.

Lewin, K. (1951) Field theory in social science: selected theoretical papers. In: Cartwright, D. (ed.) (1951). New York: Harper & Row.

Lillyman, S. (2007a) What clinical supervision means to the practitioner, patient and organisation. In: Lillyman, S. & Ghaye, T. (2007) *Effective Clinical Supervision: The Role of Reflection.* London: Quay Books.

Lillyman, S. (2007b) Action-learning sets and their place in clinical supervision. In: Lillyman, S. and Ghaye, T. (2007) *Effective Clinical Supervision: The Role of Reflection.* London: Quay Books.

Littlewood, K.A. & Strozier, A.L. (2009) Learning about leaders: exploring and measuring leadership qualities in grandparents and other relatives raising children. *Journal of Intergenerational Relationships,* **7(4):** 371–393.

Lloyd, G.C. (1996) Fostering an environment of employee contribution to increase commitment and motivation. *Empowerment in Organizations,* **4(1):** 25–28.

Luft, J. (1969) *Of Human Interaction.* Palo Alto, CA: National Press.

Martin, V., Charlesworth, J. & Henderson, E. (2010) *Managing in Health and Social Care,* 2nd edition. Oxon: Routledge.

Maslow, A. (1954) *Motivation and Personality.* New York: Harper & Row.

Maxwell, J.C. (1999) *The 21 Indispensable Qualities of a Leader: Becoming the Person Others Will Want to Follow.* Nashville: Thomas Nelson.

McCabe, C. & Timmins, F. (2006) How nurse managers let down staff. *Nursing Management,* **13(3):** 30–35.

McClelland, D.C. (1987) *Human Motivation.* Cambridge: Cambridge University Press.

McDonnell, F. & Zutshi, H. (2005) *Mapping of Leadership and Management Standards for Social Care,* 2nd edition. Leeds: Skills for Care.

McKimm, J. & Held, S. (2009) The emergence of leadership theory: from the twentieth to the twenty-first century. In: McKimm, J. & Phillips, S. (2009) *Leadership and Management in Integrated Services.* Exeter: Learning Matters.

Ministry of Health (1962) *The Ten Year Hospital Plan.* London: NHS.

Mintzberg, H. (1983) *Power In and Around Organizations.* Prentice Hall.

Morgan, G. (1996) *Images of Organization,* 2nd edition. Newbury Park, CA: Sage.

Morrison, M. (1993) *Professional Skills for Leadership: Foundations for a Successful Career.* St Louis: Mosby.

Mullins, M.J. (2005) Management and organisational behaviour. In: Barr, J. & Dowding, L. (2008) *Leadership in Health Care.* London: Sage.

Mumford, M.D., Zaccaro, S.J., Harding, F.D., Jacobs, T.O. & Fleishman, E.A. (2000) Leadership skills for a changing world: Solving complex social problems. *Leadership Quarterly,* **11(1):** 11–35.

Nevis, E.C. (1989) *Organisational Consulting: A Gestalt Approach.* New York: Gardner Press.

NHS (1990) National Health Service and Community Care Act. Available at www.legislation.gov.uk/ukpga/1990/19/introduction (accessed 25 April 2012)

NHS Confederation (1999) *Consultation: The Modern Values of Leadership and Management in the NHS*. London: NHS Confederation and Nuffield Trust.

NHS Institute for Innovation and Improvement (2005a) *NHS Leadership Qualities Framework*. Available at www.nhsleadershipqualities.nhs.uk/ (accessed 26 April 2012)

NHS Institute for Innovation and Improvement (2005b) *Managing the Human Dimensions of Change. Improvement Leaders' Guide*. Coventry: NHS Institute for Innovation and Improvement.

NHS Institute for Innovation and Improvement (2006) *NHS Leadership Qualities Framework*. Available at http://www.leadershipqualitiesframework.institute.nhs.uk/portals/0/the_framework.pdf (accessed 26 April 2012)

NHS Institute for Innovation and Improvement (2008) *Root Cause Analysis Using Five Whys*. Available at www.institute.nhs.uk/creativity_tools/creativity_tools/identifying_problems_-_root_cause_analysis_using5_whys.html (accessed 26 April 2012)

NHS Institute for Innovation and Improvement (2009) *The 360° Assessment*. Available at www.leadershipqualitiesframework.institute.nhs.uk/tabid/59/Default.aspx (accessed 26 April 2012)

NHS Wales (1998a). *Better Health: Better Wales*. Available at www.wales.nhs.uk/publications/greenpaper98_e.pdf (accessed 26 April 2012)

NHS Wales (1998b) *Putting Patients First*. Available at www.wales.nhs.uk/publications/whitepaper98_e.pdf (accessed 26 April 2012)

NHS Wales (2001) *Improving Health in Wales – A Plan for the NHS with its Partners*. Available at www.wales.nhs.uk/publications/NHSStrategydoc.pdf (accessed 26 April 2012)

NHS Wales (2011) *Together for Health*. Available at www.wales.nhs.uk/ourservices/strategies (accessed 26 April 2012)

Northouse, P.G. (2010) *Leadership. Theory and Practice*, 5th edition. London: Sage.

Owen, J. (2010) *How to Influence*. Harlow: Prentice Hall.

Parks, S.D. (2005) *Leadership Can Be Taught*. Boston: Harvard Business School Press.

Pedler, M. (1997) *Action Learning Sets in Practice*, 3rd edition. Aldershot: Gower.

Pfeffer, J. (1981) *Power in Organizations*. Marshfield, MA: Pitman Publishing.

Pfeffer, J. (1992) *Managing with Power: Politics and Influence in Organisations*. Boston: Harvard Business School Press.

Pondy, L.R. (1967) Organisational conflict: concepts and models. In: Barr, J. & Dowding, L. (2008) *Leadership in Health Care*. London: Sage.

Prochaska, J. & DiClemente, C.(2005) The transtheoretical approach. In: Norcross, J. & Goldfried, N. (2005) *Handbook of Psychotherapy Integration*, 2nd edition. New York: Oxford University Press, pp. 147–172.

Rath, T. & Conchie, B. (2008) *Strengths Based Leadership*. New York: Gallup Press.

Robbins, S.P. (1984) *Essentials of Organizational Behavior*, 3rd edition. Englewood Cliffs, NJ: Prentice Hall.

Rogers, E.M. & Shoemaker, F.F. (1971) *Communication of Innovations: A Cross Cultural Approach*, 2nd edition. New York: Free Press.

Rost, J.C. & Barker, R.A. (2000) Leadership education in colleges: toward a 21st century paradigm. *Journal of Leadership Studies*, **7(1):** 3–12.

RPA (2003) *Review of Public Administration in Northern Ireland.* Belfast: RPA.

Schein, E.H. (1985) *Organizational Culture and Leadership: A Dynamic View.* San Francisco: Jossey-Bass.

Schoemaker, P.J.H. & Russo, J.E. (1993) A pyramid of decision approaches. *California Management Review*, **36(1):** 9–31.

Scholtes, P. (1998) *The Leader's Handbook: Making Things Happen, Getting Things Done.* New York: McGraw Hill.

Schön, D. (1991) *The Reflective Practitioner: How Professionals Think in Action.* Ashgate Publishing Ltd: Farnham.

Scottish Executive (2000) *Our National Health: a plan for action, a plan for change.* Available at www.scotland.gov.uk/Resource/Doc/158732/0043081.pdf (accessed 24 April 2012)

Scottish Executive (2001a) *For Scotland's Children.* Available at www.scotland.gov.uk/Publications/2001/10/fscr (accessed 24 April 2012)

Scottish Executive (2001b) Regulation of Care (Scotland) Act 2001. Available at www.legislation.gov.uk/asp/2001/8/contents (accessed 24 April 2012)

Scottish Executive (2002) Community Care and Health (Scotland) Act 2002. Available at www.legislation.gov.uk/asp/2002/5/contents (accessed 24 April 2012)

Scottish Executive (2003) *Improving Health in Scotland – The Challenge.* Available at www.scotland.gov.uk/Publications/2003/03/16747/19929 (accessed 24 April 2012)

Scottish Executive (2005) *Building a Health Service Fit for the Future.* Available at www.scotland.gov.uk/Resource/Doc/924/0012113.pdf (accessed 24 April 2012)

Scottish Executive (2006) *Changing Lives: report of the 21st Century Social Work Review.* Available at www.scotland.gov.uk/Publications/2006/02/02094408/0 (accessed 24 April 2012)

Scottish Executive (2007) *Better Health, Better Care: Action Plan.* Available at www.scotland.gov.uk/publications/2007/12/11103453/9 (accessed 24 April 2012)

Scottish Executive (2010) *NHS Scotland Quality Strategy - putting people at the heart of our NHS.* Available at www.scotland.gov.uk/Publications/2010/05/10102307/0 (accessed 24 April 2012)

Seebohm, F. (1968) *Report of the Committee on Local Authority and Allied Personal Social Services.* London: HMSO.

Shipper, F., Hoffman, R.C. & Rotondo, D.M. (2007) Does the 360 feedback process create actionable knowledge equally across cultures? *Academy of Management Learning & Education*, **6(1):** 33–50.

Skills for Care (2008) *Leadership and Management Strategy Update 2008. Transforming Adult Social Care.* Leeds: Skills for Care.

Stanley, D. (2006) Role conflict: leaders and managers. *Nursing Management*, **13(5):** 31–37.

Stanley, D. (2009) Clinical leadership and congruent leadership. In: Bishop, V. (ed.) (2009) *Leadership for Nursing and Allied Health Professions.* Berkshire: Open University Press.

Stogdill, R.M. (1948) Personal factors associated with leadership: a survey of the literature. *Journal of Psychology*, **25**: 35–71.

Thyer, G. (2003) Dare to be different: transformational leadership may hold the key to reducing the nursing shortage. *Journal of Nursing Management*, **11(2)**: 73–79.

Timmins, F. & McCabe, C. (2005) Nurses' and midwives' assertive behaviour in the workplace. *Journal of Advanced Nursing*, **51(1)**: 38–45.

Tucker, R. (2010) An analysis of leadership qualities that influence male and female athletes in middle school interscholastic team sports. *The Sport Journal*, **13(2)**: 1.

Van Maanen, J.V. & Barley, S. (1985) Cultural organization: fragments of a theory. In: Frost, P.J., Moore, L.F., Louis, M.R., Lundberg, C.C. & Martin, J. (1985) *Organizational Culture.* Beverley Hills: Sage.

Vitello-Cicciu, J. (2001) *Leadership Practices and Emotional Intelligence of Nursing Leaders.* Unpublished dissertation. Santa Barbara, CA: Fielding Graduate Institute.

Walker, K., Berg, D. & Hildebrandt, S. (2005) *Servant Leadership: An Emergent Global Leadership Concept.* International Leadership Association Conference, Amsterdam, November 4th, 2005. Available at www.usask.ca/education/leadership/servant/survey_handout.pdf (accessed 25 April 2012)

Wall, B. (2007) Being smart only takes you so far. *Training and Development*, **January:** 64–68.

Warren, J. (2007) *Service User and Carer Participation in Social Work.* Exeter: Learning Matters.

Watson, C.M. (1983) Leadership, management and the seven keys. *Business Horizons*, **26(2)**: 8–13.

Watson, L. (2004) Self-leadership: becoming an exceptional leader. *Radiologic Technology*, **75(6)**: 457–470.

Weightman, J. (1999) *Introducing Organisational Behaviour.* Harlow: Addison Wesley Longman.

Weisinger, H. (2000) *Emotional Intelligence at Work.* San Francisco: Jossey-Bass.

Welford, C. (2002) Matching theory to practice. *Nursing Management*, **9(4)**: 7–11.

Welsh Assembly Government (2004*) Making Connections: Delivering Better Services for Wales.* Cardiff: Health and Social Care Department (Welsh Assembly Government).

Welsh Assembly Government (2005) *Designed for Life: Creating World Class Health and Social Care for Wales in the 21st Century.* Cardiff: Health and Social Care Department (Welsh Assembly Government).

Welsh Assembly Government (2007) *Strategy for Social Services in Wales over the Next Decade. Fulfilled Lives, Supportive Communities.* Cardiff: Welsh Assembly Government.

Whitmore, J. (2002) *Coaching For Performance: Growing People, Performance and Purpose*, 3rd edition. London: Nicholas Brealey Publishing.

Wong, C.S. & Law, K.S. (2002) The effects of leader and follower emotional intelligence on performance and attitude: an exploratory study. *The Leadership Quarterly*, **13**: 243–274.

Yoder-Wise, P.S. (2003) *Leading and Managing in Nursing*, 3rd edition. St Louis: Mosby.

Zilembo, M. & Monterosso, L. (2008) Nursing students' perceptions of desirable leadership qualities in nurse preceptors: a descriptive survey. *Contemporary Nurse: A Journal for the Australian Nursing Profession*, **27(2):** 194–206.

INDEX